We Walk

A volume in the series
The Culture and Politics of Health Care Work
Edited by Suzanne Gordon and Sioban Nelson

For a list of books in the series, visit our website at
cornellpress.cornell.edu.

We Walk

Life with Severe Autism

Amy S. F. Lutz

ILR Press
an imprint of Cornell University Press

Ithaca and London

First published 2020 by Cornell University Press

Printed in the United States of America

Library of Congress Cataloging-in-Publication Data

Names: Lutz, Amy S. F., 1970– author.
Title: We walk : life with severe autism / Amy S. F. Lutz.
Description: Ithaca [New York] : ILR Press, an imprint of Cornell University Press, 2020. | Series: The culture and politics of health care work | Includes bibliographical references.
Identifiers: LCCN 2020011042 (print) | LCCN 2020011043 (ebook) | ISBN 9781501751394 (cloth) | ISBN 9781501751400 (epub) | ISBN 9781501751417 (pdf)
Subjects: LCSH: Autism—Social aspects. | Autistic people—Family relationships. | Parents of autistic children.
Classification: LCC RC553.A88 L88 2020 (print) | LCC RC553.A88 (ebook) | DDC 616.85/882—dc23
LC record available at https://lccn.loc.gov/2020011042
LC ebook record available at https://lccn.loc.gov/2020011043

For Andy, Jonah, Erika, Hilary, Aaron, and Gretchen

Understanding across difference is both possible and necessary.

—*Iris Marion Young*

Contents

Preface   *ix*

Acknowledgments   *xv*

1 We Walk   *1*

2 Physical Guidance   *18*

3 Answers and Questions   *35*

4 The Next Time   *49*

5 Just Say Yes   *65*

6 All Possible Spaces   *83*

7 Praesidalism   *97*

8 The Child Who Does Not Know
   How to Ask   *115*

9 Baseline   *139*

Notes   *153*

Bibliography   *167*

Preface

I began writing about Jonah, the oldest of my five children, in 2007. *The Big Bang Theory* had recently launched, with its implicitly Aspergerian quirky genius protagonist, and the newly formed Autistic Self Advocacy Network had successfully pressured the NYU Child Study Center to end its "Ransom Notes" awareness campaign because its comparison of autism to a kidnapper portrayed the disorder in too negative a light. To me, at home with a severely autistic eight-year-old who would be hospitalized for most of the following year to stabilize his aggressive and self-injurious behaviors, the ads actually seemed pretty benign: "We have your son. We will make sure he will no longer be able to care for himself or interact socially as long as he lives. This is only the beginning . . . Autism."[1]

Today, the National Council on Severe Autism (of which I'm proud to be a founding board member) offers a definition of severe autism:

> Those who satisfy the diagnostic criteria of the DSM-5, and who, by virtue of any combination of cognitive and functional impairments, require continuous or near-continuous, lifelong services, supports, and supervision. Individuals in this category are

often nonverbal or have limited use of language, have intellectual impairment, and, in a subset, exhibit challenging behaviors, such as aggression, self-injury, and/or property destruction that interfere with safety and well-being.[2]

All I knew in 2007 was that the narrative promoted by autism rights, or neurodiversity, activists and increasingly popular media portrayals (such as Mark Haddon's award-winning novel *The Curious Incident of the Dog in the Night-Time*) looked nothing like Jonah's autism. Where were the code locks on all the exterior doors, to prevent wandering? Or the gym mats on the bedroom floor, better padded and easier to clean than the blood-stained carpet they replaced? Or the signs taped to strategic windowpanes pleading in all caps, "STOP! DO NOT HIT WINDOWS"?

Most of my articles were short, published on digital platforms like *Babble*, *Slate*, and, later, *Psychology Today*. I wrote them primarily to make severe autism visible. As an increasing number of celebrities embraced their autistic identities, such as Dan Aykroyd, Daryl Hannah, and, for a few brief days in 2014, Jerry Seinfeld, I wanted to make sure the public—particularly the policy makers Jonah will rely on for support his entire life—understood that more than 30 percent of autistic individuals are also intellectually disabled, that a third are nonverbal, and that approximately half suffer from aggressive or self-injurious behaviors.[3] And that for this population, autism isn't a difference like homosexuality, which neurodiversity advocates often compare it to, but a profound and devastating disability.

I didn't, I should clarify, write about Jonah to paint myself as a "Martyr Mommy," as self-advocate Christa Holmans describes parents such as me, who, she claims, "use their child's autism diagnosis to seek pity from others, building their entire identity around how their child being autistic has ruined their life."⁴ My primary goal has always been to capture, for those who have never known anyone like Jonah, what his severe autism looks like: a life so constrained by dangerous behaviors, processing difficulties, and a lack of abstract concepts that the most basic elements of what most of us would consider a good life are forever precluded for him: meaningful work, intimate relationships, even just the ability to independently walk out the front door and go ... anywhere.

Still, I'm puzzled by the implication that parents' stories don't also matter. Countless families are living in crisis—unable to leave the house, they spend their days hunkered down with children who are unpredictably violent, often incontinent, and may only sleep for a couple of hours each night. Unsurprisingly to this community, *Disability Scoop* reported in 2009 that the mothers of autistic adolescents and adults "experience chronic stress comparable to combat soldiers."⁵ These are parents who love their kids—who open their arms, not knowing whether they will be hugged or hit; who celebrate every accomplishment; who never stop searching for the doctors, schools, and therapists that will maximize their children's independence and overall quality of life. But they are also parents who gave up careers they loved; drained their savings accounts; neglected friendships and, too often, their other kids; and gave up vacations or even date nights because what babysitter could be left with a 150-pound fourteen-year-old who might just watch *Sesame Street* videos but who also might, in an uncontrollable rage, try to bite her arm or rip her hair out?

The pediatrician and bioethicist Lisa Freitag calls the work such parents do "extreme caregiving," which she distinguishes from typical parenting by its "complexity, prolonged duration, relentlessness, and intimacy of care."⁶ According to her conservative estimate, about a million and a half families are engaged in this labor—caring not only for children with significant intellectual and developmental disabilities, but also for medically fragile and technologically dependent kids. Despite the size of this population, Freitag has found little public discussion about extreme caregiving. In part, she attributes this to a simple lack of time for writing memoirs or even blog posts. But the bulk of the blame falls on "a cardinal rule that makes public optimism toward disability a requirement," that "effectively silences parents who speak out about the hardships they encounter"[7]—because they don't want to be mocked as "Martyr Mommies," for example.

Although Freitag focuses on parents, they aren't the only ones providing extreme care. Harvard psychiatrist Arthur Kleinman recounts his wife Joan's decade-long battle with early-onset Alzheimer's in his memoir *The Soul of Care*. As Joan's primary caregiver for most of that time, Kleinman strove to comfort her increasingly frequent agitation and aggression. He swept away the shards when she smashed picture frames and antique plates, and drove one-handed for hours so he could hold her hands to keep her from opening the car door and jumping out—stories so familiar that I couldn't suppress a running, mental commentary as I read: "Didn't they have child locks in cars in 2010? If she needs help in a public bathroom, just go in with her and dare people to complain. Taking her to the opera was probably a mistake: did you know that many venues have performances for patrons who can't sit quietly?"

Kleinman captures the sheer physical and emotional endurance of caring for someone who requires assistance in all activities of daily living, as well as round-the-clock supervision to keep her from harming herself or someone else—including those times when his endurance fails him: "Feeling helpless, I slumped to the floor, bereft of any cogent thoughts or words. Even tears wouldn't come. I felt utterly useless, unable to imagine any way to make things better. I didn't see how I could go on."[8] But he also describes moments of love, commitment, and gratitude—textbook extreme caregiving, in other words, which Freitag observes, "provides amazing highs and dangerous lows."[9]

Most importantly, Kleinman found great meaning in caregiving, which he calls "the existential activity through which we most fully realize our humanity."[10] His experience loving and caring for someone with (increasingly) severe cognitive impairment and dependency changed his entire worldview—from his own ambitions and personal relationships to his beliefs about what constitutes good medical care and, even more broadly, the purpose of government. It's not surprising, of course, that shepherding his wife through her decline and death would be so impactful—life with Jonah has transformed me also. It's impossible not to be affected by something so all-consuming. Autism in my house sometimes feels like Alice after she ate the cake in Wonderland, so big she could no longer fit through the door to the garden, only gaze at it with one enormous eye. Or maybe I'm Alice, and autism is the house I can never leave.

Perhaps the best analogy of all is that severe autism is the window, the lens that filters everything I see. The essays in this collection—including the short pieces I felt compelled to revisit and expand, as well as previously unpublished work—all wrestle with issues that changed for me once viewed through this lens. These range from deeply personal interrogations of identity, spirituality, and friendship to critical questions about the society we want to live in, the tools we need to create it, and the place of the cognitively disabled in that world.

These questions don't just concern me and Arthur Kleinman, or even the community of extreme caregivers more broadly. Care ethicists observe that care is central to all our lives, and that this private and often invisible labor is the foundation on which our society is built (as Kleinman concluded, "Care is the human glue that holds together families, communities and societies").[11] Joan Tronto argues that we need to explicitly "put responsibilities for caring at the center of [our] democratic and political agendas," adding that "if a democratic society has any commitments at all, it must have a commitment to making care—both receiving and giving care—equally and widely available to all."[12]

I consider the vision of care ethicists again in the essays "The Next Time" and "Praesidalism," but please don't ask me what the world they call for would actually look like. The fiction writer I once was would be shocked at how often my imagination has failed me since Jonah was diagnosed in 2001. But I don't think that's a bad thing. As much as our imaginations can liberate us to dream of unicorns, telekinesis, and time travel, they can also keep us from understanding lived experience very different from our own. And I don't claim to understand Jonah's experience as he lives it—that's something else I'm utterly incapable of imagining, although I'll never stop trying. But I do believe that any debate about the future—mine, my family's, my polity's—is incomplete without Jonah as I know him: contagious joy, devastating cognitive impairment, enthusiastic affection, frenetic motion, inconsolable agitation, and a total dependency that challenges our deepest assumptions about autonomy, responsibility, and citizenship.

Acknowledgments

Thanks so much to everyone who shared their experience and insight with me: Alison Singer, Bryan King, Debbie, Dominic Sisti, Hilary Lutz, Jennifer Abbanat, John Williams, Jonathan Moreno, Judith Ursitti, Karen Echols, Kevin Gray, Lester Grinspoon, Melanie, Oliver Miede, Rick Doblin, Stacey, Stephanie Lay, Susan Senator, Tara, and Tom Hibben.

Thanks to Judi Fisher for a lifetime of encouragement and to Keri Fisher for her feedback—spot on, as always.

Thanks to Suzanne Gordon and Fran Benson at Cornell University Press, who offered enthusiastic support exactly when I needed it.

Completing a manuscript while pursuing my first year of doctoral studies made for a crazy year—one that would have been impossible without the amazing support I've been so privileged to receive. Thanks to Jonah's team: Marina O'Brien, Maria Kioukis, Theresa Everett, Candace Williams, Paige Cornwell, Shaneen Brown, Ari Nugent, Emè Jackson, Chelsea Carr, Leah Okunoye, and Katie Costanza. And that doesn't even include his fabulous educators at the Preparing Adolescents and Adults for Life (PAAL) Program: Gloria Satriale, Jessica Zawicki, Lauren Erion, Ben Kaliner, Murphy Harmon, Jimmy Harrison, Matt Johnson, and Alex Richards.

Above all, thanks to my unbelievable family—my kids, Jonah, Erika, Hilary, Aaron, and Gretchen, who were always proud and never resentful (at least, they didn't show it) and my incomparable husband, Andy, who shopped and cooked and child-wrangled so I could get it all done. Never think for a moment I don't know how lucky I am.

Parts of the following essays were previously published as the following blog posts or articles: "Dear Stranger: Your Son's Autistic, Just Like Mine," *Babble*, September 13, 2007; "Where Should Special Needs Kids Be Special? Tricky Questions About How to Share Public Spaces," *Slate*, March 16, 2013; "You Do Not Have Asperger's," *Slate*, May 22, 2013; "I Don't Think That Word Means What You Think It Means," *Psychology Today*, July 29, 2016; "Bring on the 'Inspiration Porn,'" *Psychology Today*, October 19, 2016; "Presume Beneficence," *Psychology Today*, May 17, 2017; "Friends for Hire," *Psychology Today*, October 14, 2018.

Some names have been changed to protect privacy.

We Walk

1

We Walk

It's a little more than a mile from our vacation home in Gardner's Basin to the northern end of the Atlantic City boardwalk; another mile and a half to the Pretzel Factory, which now opens inconveniently at nine, although it used to open earlier. My autistic son, Jonah, walks that five-mile round trip every morning we're in Atlantic City—usually with me, sometimes with our nanny, occasionally with my husband, Andy. If they wake up early enough, one or two of his four siblings might join us for the breakfast treats they earn. But Jonah goes every day.

The streets are quiet at seven thirty, but not deserted. We pass people walking their dogs or waiting for the jitney to take them to their casino jobs. In front of the public housing project, a few men and women in baggy clothing smoke in plastic chairs. We exchange brief pleasantries. I know if I encourage Jonah to be friendly, he will simply parrot me Gracie Burns–style, "Say good morning, Jonah," so I speak for both of us. The people we pass nod and smile, but do not stare. They have seen Jonah walk by hanging on my arm or clapping his hands in front of his face until his eyes cross, or even biting his fist and squawking when he's in an uncooperative mood, and it's no longer remarkable to them.

We used to be able to cut across the park and join the boardwalk where it stretched above the ocean on wooden pilings so high that when Jonah occasionally kicked one of his flip-flops over the edge, as he was wont to do when my attention was diverted, my only option was to stick the other one in my bag and keep going. His soles are so thick and tough from his virtually lifelong aversion to shoes that he rarely got splinters. (Parenting in general, and special needs parenting especially, is about choosing your battles; I very early gave up on shoes. Jonah's much better about it now, as he is with most things, but when he was two or three I spent twenty minutes every day wrestling him into sneakers he would kick off in seconds while I wondered why it was taking so long, given the skyrocketing autism rate, for someone to invent irremovable shoes, which I imagined as little straitjackets for feet.) But that entire stretch has been closed since Superstorm Sandy accelerated the slow decay that had left the boardwalk warped and gap-toothed where there were no casinos to maintain it, sometimes with nothing but yellow tape cordoning off the missing planks. Instead we have to walk all the way down New Hampshire and up the access ramp by the incongruous oceanfront tenement that used to be turquoise but has now been painted a much less interesting shade of gray.

"No school," Jonah says frequently, while we're walking but also at other times.

"Jonah, what day is it?" I ask.

"Saturday," he says, because he always knows.

"And do we have school on Saturdays?"

"No," he says.

"That's right," I agree. "No school today or tomorrow."

Sometimes this quiets him for a while, but often the loop repeats almost immediately: "No school." I used to find the constant iterations exasperating—Jonah obviously couldn't have forgotten in the span of ten minutes the answer to a question he already knew before he asked it the first time. Now I see in this scripting a desire to engage. It's hard to know for certain, because Jonah's mind has always been stubbornly opaque to me, but I can't help but think that when Jonah starts again with "No school," what he's really saying is that he wants me to pay attention to him, that he's looking for the back and forth of conversation but doesn't know the conventions. He can't access the incredible data bank of niceties, hypothetical situations, jokes, and *Dr. Who* trivia my other kids tap into so naturally, their chatter so persistent, so demanding, that sometimes—even though I swore, in the face of Jonah's language impairment, that I would cherish every word any of my children ever uttered—I secretly wish they would, for a few minutes, just shut up. But saying "No school" triggers an exchange that is comfortable and familiar, so I say my lines with great enthusiasm and am rewarded by a squeeze from Jonah, tall enough now to put his arm around my shoulder. He nudges me until I wrap my arm around his back, and we march for a while in lockstep, like Laverne and Shirley. Just when I begin to tire of the awkward coordination necessary to keep us from tripping over each other's feet, Jonah presses his cheek against mine, hard, and I decide I could go on like this forever.

ATLANTIC CITY ISN'T the only place we walk. It's not even the most frequent place we walk. At home in Philadelphia, we hike through Valley Forge National Park and Fairmount Park, the largest city park in the world, even bigger than Central Park. We walk around the nature trail at Haverford College. If we don't have much time, we just walk around our neighbors' field or up and down our own driveway, which is harder than it sounds since it's a quarter of a mile up a steep hill. We've walked on the beach at Key Largo and down abandoned railroad tracks by the Susquehanna River in Maryland. We tried to do laps around the top deck of a cruise ship to the Bahamas last spring break but had to abort once we discovered how determined Jonah was to launch himself overboard the way he likes to jump off our little motorboat.

But Atlantic City is my favorite place to walk. I love the ocean, of course. The slow, steady exhalations of the waves inevitably quiet my ever-racing mind—a reaction so strongly conditioned I can feel my blood pressure drop as soon as we get off the expressway. And I love the wide-open mornings, walking out the front door while everyone is sleeping and not worrying about piano lessons or soccer games or birthday parties. Part of the reason we take Jonah for these long walks is that he wakes up so much earlier than the other kids, and I hate for him to spend hours fiddling with his iPad, watching bits and pieces of *Sesame Street* videos on YouTube. I know when we head out that the rest of the family won't be ready to go to the beach or out on our boat until at least ten or later, so there is no rush—if Jonah wants to stop for a few minutes, hang over the wooden rail, and watch the boys with the wetsuits and longboards that always strike me as a bit optimistic for the generally mild surf, all the better (although our leisurely pace definitely subordinates the other reason we walk: Jonah's obsession with food).

I also love the town itself. I have visited my friends in their tony shore enclaves, where tanned teenagers check your beach tags and wind chimes hang from the doorframes of charming kite shops, and they are lovely. The first vacation Andy and I took together was a weekend in Cape May, on the southern tip of New Jersey. We stayed in a bed and breakfast that had been converted from a Victorian mansion, and we rented a pedal-powered surrey and rode up and down the promenade, stopping when we got thirsty for fresh-squeezed lemonade that was gritty with the extra sugar I ordered. Now, those places make me nervous. I hover over Jonah to make sure he doesn't smear ketchup on my friends' white sofa cushions and coax him away from the floor-to-ceiling windows he likes to press his nose and lips against. I'm constantly checking that his feet aren't dirty and making sure he doesn't nonchalantly pick his nose in the middle of the homemade fudge emporium.

Atlantic City doesn't care about ketchup stains. The boardwalk is battered and sticky and cheap; there isn't much damage Jonah can do. I don't have to keep a firm grip on him, the way I do when we're in malls or restaurants. If he suddenly bolts into a store to grab something, the worst I'll be liable for is a box of Mike and Ikes. And I appreciate that people in Atlantic City don't stare when Jonah flaps his hands or when he just stops and lies face down on the ground—simply because there are much more interesting things to watch, like the woman who appears crazy and homeless and may very well be neither who is always sitting on the same bench singing gospel music; or the volunteers who troop out every morning to feed the feral cats that live under the boardwalk; even, once, a movie shoot—*The Bounty Hunter*, starring Jennifer Aniston.

But what I love most is that, despite the grime and the occasionally hilarious, always tasteless T-shirts strung like flags across every storefront, Atlantic City brims with potential. Every time Jonah and I walk past the casinos I think about the jackpots that are celebrated inside. More people, obviously, lose than win, but money can be trickled away anywhere. There are very few places where fortunes are made instantly, where people's lives are suddenly and irrevocably improved by strokes of luck. And maybe it's that combination that resonates so fiercely with me: resilience and faith, since these defined our lives for the years that Jonah suffered from random, intense rages during which he would pound himself in the face, punch through windows, and attack me and Andy as well as his teachers and aides. When I think about that time now that his behaviors have been medically stabilized, I still wonder how we persevered, managing the frequent attacks that left us bitten, bruised, and scratched; insulating Jonah's younger siblings and cousins who, thankfully, never became targets; and embracing him when the tantrums were over without (noticeably) flinching.

Actually, I know how we survived. Like the big winners in the casinos, we were lucky: we found the right doctors when we needed them, even if it sounds perverse to describe hospitalizing a nine-year-old boy for almost a year as "lucky." Still, as Jonah and I walk quickly past the Revel, since the sun bouncing off the mirrored panels of Atlantic City's newest (and already bankrupt) resort is uncomfortably hot, even so early in the morning, I haven't stopped hoping for more luck, more transformation, more miracles. Why not? Scientists have already succeeded in reversing the symptoms of Fragile X, the most common inheritable form of autism, in adult mice. I understand that we are far away from human trials, and that whatever researchers learn from these studies may be irrelevant to Jonah, who doesn't have Fragile X. But even if Jonah never benefits from this particular discovery, surely something therapeutic will emerge from the $200 million in autism research the National Institutes of Health funds every year, including studies examining the genetic, structural, and chemical impairments in autistic brains—which, when fully understood, will likely translate into new treatments for core deficits in language and socialization. If these come too late for Jonah, then at least they may ease the minds of my other kids as they plan their own families with, I imagine, significant trepidation, given the increased odds their children will be diagnosed with the disorder.

These thoughts often unspool from my mind as we pass the glassed casino entrances, catching as people go in and out a blast of air-conditioning and the frenzied chatter of slot machines (because someone is always winning in Atlantic City, even at eight thirty in the morning). I try to picture my children as adults. It's easier to do with my oldest daughter, who is already approaching my height, no longer bucktoothed and potbellied as she was when she was younger. She is the child most likely to accompany me and Jonah on our walks, and although I suspect Jonah prefers my undivided attention, he has come to really love Erika. The twins are still undifferentiated children to him—he routinely confuses their names, even though one is blonde and blue-eyed and a girl, and the other has dark eyes and hair and is a boy. But since Erika has attained the size of a grown-up, he treats her like one: listening when she warns him to keep his mitts out of the peanut butter jar, scripting with her from his favorite videos, and slipping his arm through hers as we stroll the boardwalk. For most of her life, Erika's efforts to draw with Jonah or bounce with him on the trampoline were met with consistent rejection, so I love to watch them together. "'Y Dancing' song," he might say to her, which means that he wants her to sing the mysterious phrase "Y Dancing" ("Why Dancing"?) to the tune of the *Dora the Explorer* ditty "I'm a Map"—all of which Erika understands, so she does it, causing Jonah to jump in place and clap his hands in excitement. And I think, looking at them, that my hope for remedy, for less suffering in the future, isn't unique to parents of kids with autism, or parents in general, but very possibly defines the human condition.

IF WE GET to the Pretzel Factory before nine, we have to wait. We camp out on a bench across the boardwalk, our backs to the ocean, so we can see the second the door opens.

"What's number 1?" Jonah asks.

Jonah's list making started as a way of structuring his time and letting him know how many tasks he had to complete before he could have a treat or some time with his iPad. An after-school list, for example, might look like this: (1) snack, (2) Connect Four, (3) multiplication worksheet, (4) elliptical trainer, (5) choice, and so on. But he enjoys making lists so much that he started asking for them all the time; soon we had to differentiate between "real lists" that we actually followed and "fun lists," which start off very similarly to real lists but then veer off into completely random fragments that often, but not always, include lines from *Sesame Street* videos.

"I don't know, Jonah. What is number 1?" I ask, even though I know perfectly well. But just like I would never steal the punch line of the tired jokes that have survived from my childhood to find new life in my own eager kids (What's black and white and red all over? Why is 6 afraid of 7?), I let Jonah answer.

"Walk 130 more times," he says. (The significance of "130" continues to elude me, although it pops up frequently in his lists. His number of choice used to be thirty-nine, which made sense because one of his favorite *Sesame Street* skits was a parody of the Hitchcock movie *The Thirty-Nine Steps*, during which Grover trudges up a long flight of stairs with the hope of finding something fantastic at the top—only to be met, metaphysically enough, with a brick wall. After his initial frustration, however, he finds joy sliding down the bannister, making this perhaps the best of the metaphors for life with an autistic child I constantly find in *Sesame Street*.)

"Walk 130 more times," I agree. "What's number 2?"

"Pretzel," he says. "With cheese sauce."

"As soon as they open," I say. "Do you want cream cheese or cheddar cheese?" I know the answer to this also, but so few of our conversations approach the back and forth of typical dialogue that I can't help myself.

"Cheddar cheese," he says.

"Cheddar cheese," I confirm.

The next few things on the list may be things he wants to do that day: fast boat ride, swimming, Double Shot (the most thrilling attraction at his favorite amusement pier in Ocean City), drawing with Mommy. Or he might skip right to his own idiosyncratic items.

"What's number 3?" Jonah asks.

"Number 3 is . . . ?" I respond on cue, with great anticipation.

"Jonah draws half a the, half a W and writes 'white slide,'" he says, or "Daddy, I'll be right back, walk the driveway and sit in the car," or "Coming through the window," which probably means he's thinking about another *Sesame Street* song in which chickens keep flying through a window until they fill an entire room, but who knows for sure?

I spend a lot of time wishing Jonah could tell me what he's thinking. If I had a magic pill that would make him say one thing, that's what I would want to hear. It's common for organizations trying to articulate the plight of the parents of autistic children to ask the public to imagine how they would feel if their kids could never say, "I love you," but oddly enough, that's not even in my top ten. Jonah has always shown how much he loves me: when he was very small, he had a habit of kissing me all the way up my arm that earned him the nickname Gomez (after the irrepressibly romantic *Addams Family* patriarch); if he's working with an aide and I come in to say hello, he'll jump up, grab my arm, and say, "Switch with Mommy"; when he sees me dressed for an evening out he says, "Mommy wearing the pajamas," since those flannel pants are a sure sign that I'm in for the night. It's everything else about Jonah that is so uncertain.

What does he dream about? What did it feel like when those rages used to come over him? Does he have any understanding of life and death, past and future? No, I wouldn't waste precious words to hear Jonah tell me he loves me; I'd much rather save them for something I didn't already know.

JONAH ALWAYS ORDERS the same thing: a pretzel with cheddar cheese dip and a diet peach Snapple. "Two," he says while the owner slides the pretzel into a bag, which is how I know Andy is more generous than I am when he walks with Jonah.

"One," I say firmly. This is only the beginning of a day of treats that will inevitably include a cheesesteak, french fries, and possibly fudge (which Jonah pronounces "fyooj," since that's what it looks like to him when he reads it off the box, and everyone in the family finds this so charming that instead of correcting him, we all now say it the same way).

We sit on a granite bench in the Korean War Memorial right next door, which is much more classy than anyone would expect it to be, surrounded on both sides by vendors offering hermit crabs painted like Spongebob and deep fried . . . everything, including butter, which sounds awful but must not be. Jonah wipes every last drop of cheese dip out of the plastic cup with his pretzel, while I consider the names of the New Jersey boys killed in combat. Often, Japanese tourists stroll through and pose for pictures, dwarfed by the twelve-foot bronze statue of a soldier grieving over the dog tags of his fallen friend. Their presence never fails to surprise me. I love Atlantic City, but one of the things I love most about it is that it isn't halfway across the world. The ninety-minute drive from our house in Pennsylvania is part of what makes Atlantic City so easy, and I'm not sure whether it's my age or my circumstances, but easy is all I'm after right now. I used to have quite the travel bug. Before graduate school I backpacked through Europe, Egypt, India, and Thailand; Andy and I honeymooned in China and Vietnam; and I dragged Jonah to Argentina when he was one year old because my friends invited me and I wasn't going to miss an opportunity to cross South America off my bucket list just because I had a baby in tow.

Now, I get anxious just thinking about crowded airports, long security lines, unfamiliar lodgings with doors and windows that open easily, with just a twist, and all the enticing attractions on the other side: swimming pools, beaches, amusement parks, restaurants that might seem particularly appealing to Jonah in the middle of a restless night. Still, we decided recently that his dramatically improved behavior warranted a vacation somewhere other than Atlantic City. Andy chose a Bahamas cruise that sailed from Baltimore, less than two hours away, which seemed perfect since we didn't need to fly. It was far from perfect. Jonah kept asking to jump off the ship; we had to escort him around the buffet with a tight grip so he didn't thrust his hand into a pan of mashed potatoes; he had no interest in bingo or acrobats or calypso singers. But the biggest reason we won't be going on another cruise is that Jonah's favorite day by far was the one that most closely approximated an afternoon in Atlantic City: we chartered a small fishing boat in Nassau that drove us out to a coral reef where Jonah could finally jump off 130 times—or as many times as fit in the hour we had before we needed to get back to the ship. And while at first I felt defeated, realizing that the family vacations I had always hoped we would take *someday*—camping in the national parks, churning butter in Colonial Williamsburg, ziplining in Costa Rica—really never will happen, or will happen without Jonah, by the time we made it safely back to Baltimore I had begun to wonder whether Jonah's love of the familiar was less a reflection of his developmental disability than of a strangely mature wisdom. Andy's stepfather was a merchant marine, and shortly after I met him, I asked him his favorite of the many cities he had visited. I was expecting an exotic port like Shanghai or Marseille; what he said was "Conshohocken," the town in Pennsylvania where he had lived for the past thirty years. At twenty-four, I found his attitude horribly provincial. Now, more than twenty years later, I understand what a privilege it is to be so deeply rooted. My anxiety dreams, which once featured imminent finals in courses I hadn't attended and for which I was completely unprepared, now involve moving, usually to characterless new construction, always with tremendous regret. Maybe Jonah just arrived earlier at the same epiphany that many of us come to later—not so original or uncommon, really; in fact, the exact moral of a movie Jonah has never seen, *The Wizard of Oz*: "If I ever go looking for my heart's desire again, I won't look any further than my own back yard. Because if it isn't there, I never really lost it to begin with."[1]

I think a lot about happiness while we walk, mostly because Jonah is so happy and it makes me happy to watch him: laughing not because he is amused, but because he is joyous. It's completely obvious from his unselfconscious yelps, his huge smile, and his hard hugs that for him, at this moment, the world is perfect, and I'm grateful yet again that I'm able to give my son countless weekends at this place about which he loves every single thing: swimming, boating, eating, walking, rotating through amusement piers and water parks from Atlantic City to Wildwood. When you have a child with a profound disability, all those dreams you had before he was born coalesce into just one, since without happiness there is no quality of life. Before Jonah's mood was medically stabilized, he would cycle through violent tantrums, disconsolate weeping, and maniacal laughter several times a day, his affect reflecting nothing but his screwy neurochemistry. And he wasn't the worst: on the Neurobehavioral Unit at the Kennedy Krieger Institute in Baltimore, where Jonah was hospitalized for ten months while doctors struggled to control his rages, there were children who would spend all day punching themselves in the face, hundreds of times an hour; or sit motionless, completely disengaged from everything and everyone around them, even their own parents.

But loving a disabled child also makes you realize why happiness, although vital, isn't enough. It feels like it should be: How many people, including the neurotypical population, can say they want only what they already have? For Jonah, a loop on a roller coaster, a splash in the ocean, a box of markers, and a soft pretzel (with cheese sauce) are all he needs to be genuinely happy. Why doesn't that make him the luckiest person on the planet? Am I guilty of projecting onto my son my own desires for romantic love, for friendship, for creative and intellectually stimulating work that makes a difference in the world—for self-actualization just as Abraham Maslow described it in the pyramid taught in every Psych 101 textbook?

I'm not going to argue that some kinds of happiness are better than others, because that's not the main thing I worry about when I consider Jonah's future. The real problem is that his happiness will always be dependent on factors over which he has little control. He will always need someone to drive him to Atlantic City or buy him a pretzel or take the time to sit down and make a fun list with him. And that makes me sick inside, the fear that someday—his parents gone, his four siblings well-intentioned yet scattered, perhaps, or overwhelmed with their own lives—Jonah may be stuck in a residential placement with aides who have no idea what he means when he says "Double Shot 130 more times," and no inclination to find out.

I have friends who also worry about the happiness of their disabled children, but for different reasons. Their kids, unlike Jonah, are high functioning enough to recognize their differences from typical peers and to want what they want—prom dates, driver's licenses, college. I listen to my friends describe the inappropriate behavior, the rejection, the mortification of their other children, and still I would swap with them in an instant, even if Jonah's increased capabilities not only made him no happier, but also left him struggling with frustration, yearning, and poor self-esteem. At least then Jonah would have some agency in the world. He would be able to get on a train by himself if he decided he wanted to stroll the boardwalk on a beautiful summer day. Or maybe he would choose to live in Atlantic City. He could stay in our shore house and walk to work at the Pretzel Factory, which, unlike many boardwalk businesses, is open year-round. How perfect would that be? The Pretzel Factory churns out thousands of pretzels a day—for corporate catering, for schools, for retail. They would never miss the two or three or eight pretzels Jonah would simply consider perks of the job. After work, he could stop at his favorite pizzeria, Tony Baloney's, for a cheesesteak if he wanted to treat himself, or take the jitney straight home and fix a plate of sliced turkey and dates he could eat while watching videos on the computer. I think, for Jonah, that would be a good life.

THE WALK BACK from the Pretzel Factory is often more challenging, since the shops are open and Jonah knows exactly which ones stock the best flavors of Mike and Ikes. But I know also, and as we approach his favorite dollar store I position myself between him and the entrance, with its table strewn with sunglasses that I have picked over many times, since I find sunglasses impossible to hold on to and so spend as little on them as possible. I have, in the past, encouraged Jonah to wear sunglasses, since the sun is especially bright in this direction, and I still believe he would be more comfortable, but he always refuses: "No glasses."

Sometimes as we trudge home, Jonah dragging hot and heavy on my arm, I imagine teaching him to run, my favorite form of exercise. I no longer run the crazy distances I covered while training for the 2011 Philadelphia marathon, but I still run four or five miles several times a week, and it's fun to think about Jonah and me training together for a 5K. It's appealing to consider how his fitness would improve, and how meaningful it would be to share such an important part of my life with Jonah when so many other parts are inaccessible to him. But then I wonder whether Jonah would have been too tired and breathless to tell me a joke had we been running that amazing day last summer when he turned to me with a big smile on his face and said, "She dreams about goats."

I blinked at him for half a second, recognizing immediately what he was talking about but stunned at his obvious intention. Earlier that morning, while he was waiting for me to lace up my sneakers, Jonah had repeatedly played a sketch from *Elmo's World* about a girl who loves books. She loves them so much she wears a book for a hat and books for shoes. She sleeps on a bed made of books in a house made of books. Once her passion has been firmly established, the narrator asks, "Do you know what she dreams about?"

Rabbits!

"I love rabbits, too," the girl announces. The end.[2]

I've often been able to amuse Jonah by deliberately garbling the words to *Sesame Street* videos. But this was the first time Jonah, without any prompting, misquoted one to me. He knew very well the girl didn't dream about goats. He was trying to be funny.

"Goats!" I said. "She didn't dream about goats. She dreamt about . . . peanut butter!"

"Yes," Jonah said happily.

"No, you know she didn't," I said.

"Elephants," he said. We went back and forth the entire trip to the Pretzel Factory: fish, boats, puppies, boots, cars, markers, ketchup. "That's what you probably dream about, Jonah: ketchup!" I said. We were both laughing. It was the most magical exchange I ever had with my son, and we haven't shared another one like it all winter. Sometimes I'll ask, "What does the girl who loves books dream about, Jonah? Does she dream about light bulbs?" Sometimes he might even say, "Yes," and grin, but he doesn't offer any substitutions of his own.

Much has been written recently exalting mindfulness, or living in the moment—including obvious benefits, like stress relief, and others that aren't so intuitive, like staving off colds and improving military performance. And while I'm sure that mindfulness would in fact help me sleep better and lose weight, I'm just not very good at it—which I suspect puts me in the significant majority, since if mindfulness were easy and natural, entire books wouldn't have been written about how to achieve it. While being a product of our frenetic culture is certainly cause enough, I discovered during a bioneurofeedback assessment that my neurological wiring particularly predisposes me against mindfulness. After attaching sensors to my scalp and monitoring my response to various computer tasks, the doctor pronounced me deficient in theta waves, the slow brain waves accessed during meditation. Although I had gone into the test secretly suspecting that bioneurofeedback was just high-tech quackery, the results were surprisingly insightful. I am incapable of napping and being hypnotized; I don't enjoy jigsaw puzzles or fishing or sprawling on the beach. My mind is never quiet.

Except during these slow, expansive mornings with Jonah, the hours drained of everything extraneous so all that remains is the sun, the ocean, and the two of us—all moving gently along our predictable paths. I tell Jonah what day it is, and I tell him again. We entwine our fingers as we watch the fishing boats that dock across the inlet from our house heading out to sea and the shopkeepers setting out their plastic beach toys and racks of cheap sundresses. If my mind wanders briefly to an email I need to write or a poker hand I played the night before, Jonah always calls me back: "What's number 1?" No wonder these walks inspire Jonah to push his limits. Call it magic, call it mindfulness—just other ways to describe a focused engagement uncompromised by YouTube and DVDs, phone calls and texts, kids, school, work, chores, rushing, driving, planning. Who doesn't stretch and unfurl under that brilliant light, the undivided attention of the beloved?

It's taken me a while to relinquish my deeply ingrained hierarchies: running over walking; sweat and exertion over quiet companionship; speed and distance and heart rate over simply putting one foot in front of the other. Maybe someday Jonah may decide, on his own, that it's time to pick up the pace. But until then, we walk.

2

Physical Guidance

Ever notice how often we ask people to do things when in fact we are actually telling them? We might ask our spouses, for example, "Do you mind walking the dog before you go to work?" or say to our children, "How about if you take a shower before bed?" And our spouses and our children generally do what we request, because they know we aren't really asking.

I only noticed this when I observed how often Jonah's aides asked him to do whatever was next on his schedule: "Are you ready to go for a walk?" they might say, or, "Why don't you go get Big Boggle?" Since Jonah doesn't understand this courtesy, he would often reply, "No walk," or "No Big Boggle."

"We want to reward appropriate language use, so if you ask him to do something and he says no, we should honor it," I explained to the aides. "Please don't ask him to do something if he doesn't really have a choice."

Jonah's life could, not inaccurately, be described as an endless onslaught of impositions. From the earliest age, much of what he learned was difficult and contested, as it is for most severely autistic children: speaking, toilet training, table manners, basic academic skills like matching, sorting, and building—all these required endless hours of practice, punctuated by Jonah's hysterical protests. It's hard to guess at his hierarchy, or whether he even had one; haircuts, dentists, speech therapy, even simply being asked by his teacher to complete an easy puzzle or color a worksheet, all elicited indistinguishable rages. But without a doubt for me the hardest to watch was when we took Jonah to the feeding clinic at the Children's Hospital of Philadelphia (CHOP) and forced him to eat.

IN AUGUST 2002, JONAH was three years old and ate nothing but pretzels smeared with peanut butter. We blended bananas, ice cream, protein powder, fiber, and liquid vitamins into a noxious gray shake that he willingly drank twice a day, so he wasn't particularly malnourished, but it was also clear this wasn't a tenable situation. When he was one, Jonah ate almost everything. By eighteen months, it seemed like he rejected something new each week—Andy and I used to joke about which food had been most recently "voted off the island," *Survivor*-style. It didn't make sense that he had actually stopped liking these foods, some of which, like french fries, had been tremendous favorites, or that they somehow suddenly triggered the sensory sensitivities that are so prevalent in autism. Perhaps his extreme selectivity was, as some experts posit, part of an overall regression that many autistic kids experience between the ages of one and two. Or maybe it was a manifestation of his need for control over his environment—a popular explanation for all kinds of intransigence exhibited by kids with and without disabilities. Regardless, it was clear we needed professional help before Jonah refused the pretzels as well. Fortunately, one of the best pediatric hospitals in the country was only half an hour away. They offered a month-long, full-time outpatient feeding program that required Jonah to take all his meals in the hospital. I grabbed the first available opening.

We arrived the first day by eight-thirty in the morning and proceeded to the third floor, where Jonah was weighed and measured.

At thirty-three pounds, he was perfectly average for his age. This was typical for autistic patients, who represented approximately half the hundred or so children admitted to the day program every year. Their problems had less to do with the amount of food they consumed than with variety of diet: during my stay I heard about a child who ate just coffee cake and grapes, another who ate cranberry applesauce and one particular brand of hot dog. One boy would only eat in the backyard, wearing just a diaper, with the garden hose running.

I knew from my first inquiries that virtually all the kids who finished the program ended up closer to their goals. Granted, sometimes those goals were very modest. Some of the patients had, for various reasons, been fed through tubes their entire lives. There appears to be a critical period for learning to eat in the first year of life, and children who never have the opportunity to chew and swallow can lose those natural instincts. Simply learning to take a bite of applesauce off a spoon might be a tremendous victory for them, and repeated stays in the day program might be necessary for anything approaching typical eating habits to emerge.

Autistic kids, I was told, who don't have these medical issues, were typically discharged with a greatly expanded diet of twenty or more foods. But almost every one of these transformations required the use of physical guidance—a technical term for a very controlled kind of force-feeding. As we were introduced to Don, Rebecca, and Elisa, the feeding therapists, I couldn't help but wonder which one of them would hold Jonah down, which one would force the food into his mouth. It was hard to imagine. They all seemed so young and nurturing.

Not that physical guidance was the first step. For the first four days, the team tried to coax Jonah to eat using positive reinforcement. Actually, since there was no real food involved, "eat" is a stretch. I had no idea how thorough the protocol would be. While I watched through a one-way mirror, Don began with a dry spoon, guiding Jonah hand-over-hand until he put it in his mouth and then placed it back on his plate. At first, Jonah cried and struggled, but it was the same level of objection he routinely raised to having his diaper changed or having his teeth brushed, so it wasn't that difficult to watch. After all, he wasn't being forced to ingest anything.

Each time Don managed to slip the spoon in his mouth, Jonah was rewarded with a few seconds of play. Out of a big box of toys, he chose an electronic talking Winnie-the-Pooh toy with letter and number buttons he could push. It was a perfect prize for him: like many autistic kids, Jonah was hyperlexic, obsessed with letters and numbers. This strategy seemed to work. By the end of the second day, he was picking up the spoon and putting it in his mouth completely on his own. On the third day, Don started dipping Jonah's spoon in apple juice, which he didn't even seem to notice. He was so enthralled with the Winnie-the-Pooh toy that he walked right into the treatment room and allowed himself to be buckled into a Rifton chair, a child-size restraining seat with a desktop that snaps on to the armrests. But these early successes left me with no illusions. Although more than half the clinic's patients responded to this reward system, I knew going in that Jonah wouldn't be one of them. Many of those kids were recovering from untreated reflux or food allergies, learning for the first time in their lives that food didn't have to make them sick. Jonah didn't have these medical issues. If there was anything in the world compelling enough to make him eat, I would have found it. Bribing him with letters and numbers was one of the first things we tried.

Although I couldn't help but be impressed by how slowly and deliberately the team executed the treatment plan, I also never lost the feeling we were acting out an elaborate charade—one that we all knew would fail. Sure enough, when the team introduced applesauce during the last meal on the third day, Jonah threw a huge tantrum. Still, the team wasn't ready to give up on less intrusive strategies—although the coordinator of the day program, Rachel, did restrain Jonah from behind while a therapist tried to slip the spoon between his teeth, something she was only successful in doing a couple of times. Behind the one-way mirror, my face twisted with the effort of holding back tears. I couldn't imagine what Jonah must be thinking: strapped into a chair, alone in a tiny room with strangers trying to shove a slime-covered spoon into his mouth. To me, it seemed like the kind of experience that could traumatize a child for life. This worry had so preoccupied me in the weeks leading up to Jonah's admission that I had called Rachel to ask whether any patients had ever been so psychologically damaged by their stay at the feeding clinic that they stopped eating altogether. She assured me this had never happened. As troubled as I was by Jonah's peanut butter and pretzel diet, it was certainly better than a feeding tube. One of the other parents in the day program, Larry, had graphically described for me life with a toddler who wouldn't eat: when his son spit his feeding tube out, as frequently occurred, Larry had to force it back down his throat.

After the first applesauce session, Rachel called Jonah "one of the best disrupters" she had seen in a long time. The next day, he became even more efficient in his protests, crying and flailing significantly less and simply clenching his jaw. Since the team still wasn't using physical guidance, this was highly effective. Don was able to sneak the spoon in his mouth in fewer than half the trials during all three meals. Surprisingly, once it was in his mouth, Jonah didn't seem to mind the taste of the applesauce. He didn't wipe his tongue, as I'd seen him do after eating something he didn't like, or scream or carry on. He quieted immediately and played with his Winnie-the-Pooh toy.

Finally, at the end of the fourth day, Don met me in the lounge to talk while Jonah watched a video. It was time to decide: the therapists were ready to start physical guidance, if I agreed. Don wanted me to know, however, that there was another type of protocol that didn't require any force. Called nonremoval of the spoon, this methodology involved presenting food to the child and simply holding it in front of his face until he accepted it. This obviously could take a long time; although the therapists in the day program rarely followed this protocol, Rachel told me about one case in which a single meal lasted six hours. Studies indicated that both nonremoval of the spoon and physical guidance were equally effective over the long run—although, interestingly, nonremoval of the spoon was associated with more negative vocalizations.

I thought for a minute. What I wanted to ask Don was, Which did he think was worse, the death penalty or life in prison? Jonah obviously wouldn't enjoy either of these alternatives. The faster gains made by using physical guidance held a lot of appeal. I recognized, as I told Don that he could start physical guidance on Monday, that I wasn't just considering what was best for Jonah. As much as I didn't want Jonah trapped in a Rifton chair all day, I myself didn't want to sit behind that one-way mirror watching the entire stand-off. It made me feel slightly better when Don confirmed that nearly all the parents presented with the same choice opted for physical guidance, but I still wondered. Was that because we're all basically selfish, or because physical guidance really involved less suffering?

I KNOW I HAVE an extreme, unqualified faith in experts. Not only do I trust them completely, but I'm most pleased when they tell me what to do without consulting me first. I suspect they are just trying to be courteous when they present me with choices and solicit my preferences, but—as I readily admit—I have absolutely no idea whether a tree leaning over my driveway should be cut down, whether I should replace all four tires or just the bald rear ones, or whether my younger son needs glasses. I'm sure this makes me an easy mark. But my fear of being wrong eclipses any concern I have about being exploited.

Looking back, I think I can locate the origin of this faith in the moment when Don asked me whether I thought the team should start using physical guidance. I have a terrible memory, but I remember that meeting so well, particularly my sense of bewilderment. Why were these trained medical professionals even asking me? If I knew how to make Jonah eat, we wouldn't be here. I couldn't imagine telling them how best to do their jobs.

Many parents feel differently, I know. While we were at the feeding clinic, I heard that one mother had recently withdrawn her child because she was unhappy with the program. I was stunned. What, I kept wondering, would she do instead? There was no more respected, or more effective, facility for treating kids with feeding problems than CHOP.

I never spoke with that mother or her son. Perhaps his condition was not as urgent as those of the other outpatients I had met, so she didn't feel she was compromising his safety. One thing I've come to understand—a corollary, if you will, of my faith in experts—is that skepticism is a luxury. The bigger the problem, it seems, the fewer solutions you have to address it. Of all the different types of privilege that have enabled Jonah to make so much progress, perhaps the most important was our access to the best experts in the field. Once you've found them, once you've secured their help, you have to trust them. Now, I know there is a name for this reliance on others' knowledge: epistemic dependence. And I've read the philosopher John Hardwig's argument that "because the layman is the epistemic inferior of the expert . . . rationality sometimes consists in refusing to think for one-self."[1] But in 2002, I didn't need graduate school to know that we really had no alternative. There's nothing on the other side of the CHOPs of the world but a terrifying abyss.

BY OUR FIFTH day at the feeding clinic, I stopped using the term *force-feeding*. The members of the team were very sensitive and corrected me every time I used it. Force-feeding as they had seen it done in the home was a far more brutal enterprise than what occurred in the day program. Parents, without the equipment or the technique necessary to properly restrain a child, sometimes lay down on their children, using their full body weight as leverage. They pushed food into their children's mouths until they choked on it. The most traumatizing thing for the victims of such efforts was the parental anger and frustration that inevitably precipitated the force-feeding in the first place. Emotional scars sometimes left the children with worse feeding problems than they started with.

Physical guidance, in contrast, was much more structured and controlled. Don recited the rules for Jonah, as he did at the beginning of each meal—only now the rules included, "If you don't take a bite, I'm going to help you, like this," at which point Don gripped his own jaw to show Jonah what he meant. Not that he understood, yet. But I knew the point of this repetition was that, after a few meals, Jonah would know that he was expected to abide by certain conditions.

Don presented the first spoonful of applesauce with the directive "Jonah, take a bite." Jonah refused, as usual. Next, Don tried to feed Jonah. When he still wouldn't accept the spoon, Rebecca held his arms by his side while Don applied gentle pressure to his jaw to open his mouth.

This was where the feeding team's qualifications and distinctions fell apart for me. No layperson in the world wouldn't have considered this force-feeding. Jonah was restrained, his mouth opened, and food inserted until he swallowed it. Still, the first session wasn't as bad as I thought it would be. It was actually very similar to previous meals. Jonah cried when the applesauce was presented, but as soon as it was in his mouth and Don and Rebecca released him, he was happy again. From my vantage point, it seemed like Don used increasingly less force, barely touching Jonah, until the last trial, when Jonah opened his mouth on his own. He wasn't hysterical between trials, and he didn't desperately try to get out of the Rifton chair. I thought he was probably more agitated when Don first introduced the dry spoon. Afterward, I observed Jonah as we passed the hours until "lunch" running around the rooftop playground and watching *Sesame Street* videos in the lounge. He didn't seem depressed at all. Maybe I shouldn't have been so surprised: Jonah never was one to hold a grudge.

The second session went even better: Jonah only required physical guidance in three out of fifteen trials. The other times he opened his mouth on his own, even though there was a lot more applesauce on the spoon than when it was first introduced. Granted, he still didn't want to take his bites—he wouldn't pick up the spoon voluntarily, and he did cry and try to turn his head away, but once Rebecca put her hand on his forehead and he saw that resistance was futile, he opened his mouth. Don and Rebecca agreed that Jonah liked the applesauce; Rebecca told me that during one trial a little bit escaped out of the corner of his mouth and Jonah flicked out his tongue and licked it up.

He did even better during the last meal of the day, requiring physical guidance on only two trials. More importantly to the therapists, there were a few trials where Jonah didn't cry at all, just agreeably opened his mouth and ate his applesauce. The forms Don filled out during every session tracked negative vocalizations as well as other disruptive behaviors, so the decreased crying was very significant. I called Andy at work as soon as I pulled out of CHOP's parking garage. I told him that I wasn't even allowed to bring peanut butter and pretzels the next day, because Jonah would be eating at least two ounces of applesauce at each session, the amount gradually increasing until he reached the goal of seven ounces of food per meal. I reported that the therapists would immediately start introducing new foods, alternating the applesauce with bites of yogurt. And, for the first time since we started the program, I let myself describe the family dinners I always wanted to have. We considered our friends' various traditions. My favorite was my tennis partner's: everyone goes around the table reporting the best and worst things that happened that day. Even the fact that Jonah couldn't talk didn't discourage me.

Over the next two days, Jonah not only accepted yogurt, but also began feeding himself with the spoon. Don and Rebecca were thrilled with his progress, and of course, so was I. It's hard to keep your expectations from spiraling when one success is continually followed by another, and I sailed into the observation room for the last feeding session on our seventh day excited to see Jonah eat solid food for the first time. The apple Don cut into tiny pieces seemed practically indistinguishable from the applesauce Jonah ate willingly the meal before.

But it was distinguishable to Jonah, who became hysterical as soon as he saw it on the spoon. Although he had always swallowed the applesauce and yogurt once it was in his mouth, he spit out the apple. The physical guidance protocol required Don to replace the apple immediately, so Jonah's disruptive behaviors weren't rewarded, but Jonah pushed it out again with his tongue. A CHOP psychologist observing the session told me that she had seen therapists sitting for two hours or more, pushing food back into a child's mouth as fast as it was spit out. Jonah only took ten minutes to swallow one bite of apple—but that still translated into about fifty attempts.

It was nearly impossible to watch. This was the level of invasiveness that had bothered me from the beginning, and although I knew this was the only thing left that would get Jonah to eat, part of me felt like rushing in and rescuing him. Watching the physical guidance with the applesauce and yogurt hadn't bothered me, because it was obvious that Jonah really did like them. He didn't seem to like the apple, however, at times even gagging on it (Don told me later that the gagging was his fault, because he pushed the apple piece far back into Jonah's mouth, hoping to initiate a swallowing reflex). On a few of the trials, Jonah chewed a couple of times, causing Don and Rebecca (and me, behind the mirror) to erupt into cheers, but then he always spit the apple out.

The next morning, I drove into the city filled with dread, anticipating three very long meals: Jonah spitting out the apple until it deteriorated into unrecognizable pulp and was replaced with a fresh piece, over and over again. And that was how the first trial of the morning proceeded. Jonah had to be fed the apple twenty times before he swallowed it, but he took the yogurt and applesauce used to round out the rotation without incident, which made me smile. In his position, I would have rejected everything Don offered me after such a profound betrayal.

On the second trial, Jonah ate the apple after only three attempts. Behind the mirror, I cheered so loud that Don and Elisa heard me in the treatment room. Could Jonah possibly have come around so fast?

In fact, that brief protest was the last one of any significance during our entire stay. It was as if a switch had been thrown in Jonah's head. The next time the apple was presented, he ate it— just like he ate the pear he was offered at lunch and the cantaloupe Don introduced at dinner. Everyone was shocked, including the therapists. Not that they had any doubts Jonah would eat those foods, eventually. They just hadn't thought it would happen so quickly.

Over the next week, Jonah accepted new foods at every meal: pasta, waffle, carrot, chicken, egg. Occasionally, he complained, but he never required physical guidance at more than one trial before he started eating on his own. Andy, our nanny Marina, and I were all trained as feeders, and when we started using the protocol at home, the transition went smoothly. We bought a Rifton chair of our own, which we set up in a quiet corner of the breakfast room. Although we had to use physical guidance a few times during the first meal, Jonah quickly learned that the rules that applied at the day program also applied in our kitchen.

Just before our discharge, I made a discovery that even a week earlier would have instigated a major crisis. The pretzels that, for the past six months, had made up the core of Jonah's diet were actually made of soy, since he was on a gluten- and casein-free diet at the time. This was long before Whole Foods and Trader Joe's began carrying a wide selection of gluten-free items, so I typically ordered them directly from the manufacturer. When I opened my last bag, I called the company, only to be told that the pretzels were completely out of stock and would be for the next two to three weeks. I couldn't even imagine how long Jonah would have refused to eat if we had run out before his admission to the feeding clinic.

Instead, it felt less like a catastrophe and more like a sign from God: the era of peanut butter pretzels was finally over.

BITTER OPPOSITION HAS been and continues to be raised against the use of force in autism treatment, but these debates more typically unfold in a different context from physical guidance: the use of applied behavior analysis (ABA). ABA is a popular system of data-based instruction used to teach autistic children many different kinds of skills, as well as to replace inappropriate or dangerous behavior. The Kennedy Krieger Institute, where Jonah was inpatient for almost all of 2008, reports that "over a thousand studies reporting on ABA-based assessment and treatment techniques have been published since the 1960s" and notes that such protocols successfully "reduce problem behavior and increase appropriate skills for individuals with intellectual disabilities (ID), autism, and related disorders."[2] The initial protocol followed by the feeding team—breaking down a task (eating) into small, discrete steps (like accepting a dry spoon)—is classic ABA.

But opponents, like Michelle Dawson, argue that the purpose of ABA is to turn "autistic children into robots or trained seals." She blasts "the autism-ABA industry [for] enhanc[ing] then exploit[ing] the non-autistic horror and dread of autism and autistics," and claims "parents and their industry have marketed autistics as worthless agents of personal, social, and financial destruction."[3] A fellow self-advocate, who blogs under the pseudonym Birdmad Girl, worked as an ABA technician herself and now considers it "abuse": "To ABA, an autistic person is nothing more than the unruly embodiment of behaviors to be reinforced, shaped, or extinguished, a list of 'excesses' and 'deficits' to be tallied and managed. A defiant child to be made compliant. Basically, I was a glorified dog trainer." She concludes, "It is a real challenge to find any adult who was subjected to this 'therapy' as a child who does not now have PTSD."[4]

These are hardly fair critiques of ABA as a field. As practitioners like Peter Gerhardt point out, ABA includes a tremendous range of teaching strategies united primarily by their emphases on replication and data collection.[5] However, it is true that Jonah, like many severely autistic children, spent many hours when he was younger undergoing the kind of repetitive drilling that Dawson and Birdmad Girl find so torturous. I obviously know nothing about the adults with PTSD Birdmad Girl references. But they are apparently articulate enough to describe their experiences, which suggests they don't have the profound deficits that both prevent many autistic children from learning in less structured environments and correlate with better responses to ABA than those who are more mildly impaired.[6] My friends credit ABA with teaching their autistic kids to wash their hands, get dressed, tolerate dental cleanings, and prepare their own meals. Most importantly, they report increased communication skills. One mom notes that her daughter now has "literally hundreds of nouns and verbs that she can fluently use to request items/activities." Alison Singer, president of the Autism Science Foundation, told me, "The most valuable improvement came when Jodie learned 'first/then.' Through this program she learned to wait for things, and to complete a less preferred task before moving on to a preferred task. Life changing!"[7]

Such a simple construction: first/then. First you take a shower, then you watch your iPad. First we eat breakfast, then we go to the beach. It took Jodie six months of hard work before she finally understood.

If the divide between autistic self-advocates like Michelle Dawson and Birdmad Girl and parents of severely autistic children like

Alison and myself breaks down to one thing, it's this: self-advocates assume there's an easier way. Alison and I know there isn't.

Fourteen years later, I'm sure Jonah doesn't even remember the feeding clinic. Now, we have a different problem: regulating his appetite. He loves almost all foods—except bananas, which have been mysteriously aversive for him since he was a preschooler, when he would actually fly into a rage at the sight of one. Interestingly, he has always liked the taste of bananas, which composed the bulk of the shakes we made to supplement his peanut butter and pretzel diet, and he asks, unironically, for banana bread whenever I bake it. His kindergarten teachers carried bananas around the classroom, trying to desensitize him, and maybe that helped somewhat, since the worst he does now is say, "No banana," whenever someone eats one in his general proximity. But we don't make him eat them—we don't need to, now that he happily eats many fruits and vegetables, along with all meats, cheeses, and starches. Jonah, honestly, has a broader diet than I do.

It's certainly possible that Jonah would have outgrown his extreme pickiness on his own, even without the feeding clinic. Many of his earlier issues are now resolved—either because we've successfully stabilized his mood, or because of increased exposure or years of patient instruction or maybe just because, like all kids, he's matured a lot. He doesn't draw *Sesame Street* characters on the walls anymore, or flush his electronic devices down the toilet when they need to be charged. He no longer fights against haircuts or blood draws or even, when I think back, about the thing he hated the most as a toddler: wearing shoes.

But I'm not sorry we didn't wait to see whether Jonah would start eating on his own, because his experience at the feeding clinic does not seem to have traumatized him. Not only does he eat more foods than I ever imagined he would, but his cooperation across all medical settings indicates that he doesn't find them aversive. (Anyone who has ever seen Jonah's agitation at the mere mention of the word "tickle"—"No tickle! No tickle!"—can confirm that he is emphatic in his refusals.) In fact, none of the intense interventions we pursued—decisions some of my friends and family members doubted they would ever be able to make—netted anything but positive, even transformative, results: hospitalizing Jonah for almost a year, pursuing electroconvulsive therapy, and of course physical guidance. I'm not sure why Jonah wasn't scarred by any of these experiences, but I have a few theories. I believe in human resilience. I believe in luck. And I haven't ruled out the possibility that intent matters: that evidence-based interventions guided by love and delivered to those in desperate need are rarely traumatizing in the way similar actions might be under very different circumstances—despite what Birdmad Girl might believe. Jonah didn't enjoy the physical guidance, obviously, but I'm also certain he didn't find it as invasive as, for example, political prisoners force-fed to end hunger strikes. Of course, I can't rule out that the intellectual and developmental disabilities that ultimately necessitated these treatments prevented Jonah from processing them the way a typical person might. Assessing the feeding clinic, like so much else, comes back to the gulf forever separating me from my son: I'll never really know what he knows, or how he interprets it.

I focus on outcomes: physical guidance was an unqualified success. So much so that, before Jonah's discharge, Rachel explained to me how the three-step compliance method—of which physical guidance is one example—can also be used to teach very young children of any ability level many different skills, such as dressing, brushing teeth, or cleaning up. "First, give a verbal cue, such as 'Pick up your toy,'" she explained. "Then, model the desired action yourself. Finally, help the child pick up the toy by guiding him hand-over-hand." But I never did try it with my other kids. Instead, I asked, I reasoned, I reminded—occasionally I bribed, and frequently I yelled. Now, when I see how far Jonah has come, I can't help but wonder: What might my other children have accomplished, if only I had forced them to do it?

3

Answers and Questions

I will never forget Ben—even though, in many ways, I already have. I can't remember what he looked like, beyond the sweet, round softness common to all toddlers. I can't even remember his real name. I suppose it's not that surprising: I only saw him once, twelve years ago, in a make-up music class my sister Keri and I took my then year-old twins and her sixteen-month-old son to after missing our typical day because of a family vacation. But I will never forget how Ben spun wildly to the music and ran in happy circles around the room. He didn't follow along with the teachers like the other kids. Sometimes he dropped into his mother's lap for a hug, but he wouldn't come when she called him. Watching him was like watching Jonah at music class when he was two, when I still thought he spent most of the class playing with the window blinds because he just wasn't as interested in music as my friend's daughter. Even Keri recognized the signs; when Ben started vocalizing in the same consonant-free, almost shrieky way we often heard from Jonah, she leaned over to me and whispered, "Spectrum?"

"Definitely," I whispered back. Then, "Do you think I should say something?"

"No," Keri said emphatically. Maybe, she added, the mother already knew.

But it was clear the mother didn't know. I had overheard one of the music teachers observing that Ben reminded him of his own son, now grown, who had ADHD. "Don't say that," Ben's mother laughed nervously. That's why I was so sure. To mothers of autistic children, an ADHD diagnosis would be nothing, a minor bump in the developmental road they would swap for in a heartbeat. Kids with ADHD grow into young people who go to college, pursue careers, live independently, get married, and have families. Kids with autism have indeterminate futures; they may one day do some of these things. More likely, they won't.

Keri was so alarmed at the possibility I might approach Ben's mother that in the end, I didn't say anything. After spending more of the class watching her and her son than I did watching my own babies, trying to decipher whether the sadness I thought I saw on her face was a projection of my own concern or the nascent realization that her son wasn't like the other children in the class, I just left. Ben was twenty months old, I had found out. He would be back to the doctor for his two-year checkup in four months. Surely his pediatrician would notice such a classic constellation of symptoms and refer his mother to a specialist for an evaluation, I reassured myself.

How do I know that's what I was thinking, or the brief words Keri and I exchanged, when I can't even remember what color hair Ben had? Because I wrote about this episode, right after it happened.[1] In 2007, I was thirty-seven. I had been a fiction writer my whole life: from the illustrated tale of a witch and a pumpkin I wrote when I was three to my impassioned tenures on the editorial boards of my high school, then my college literary magazines, to my master of fine arts degree from Indiana University. I wasn't hugely successful by any means, but I had published many stories and poems in small, prestigious journals; I had even procured an agent for a novel draft I had recently completed. Yet, somehow, I was losing my taste for fiction. For the first time in my life, it struck me as . . . indulgent. Jonah was eight years old. He had already been kicked out of our in-district autistic support class after breaking a teacher's nose. None of the doctors we saw, none of the medications we tried, stabilized his behavior for very long. How could fiction ease my fear that someone was going to get hurt, perhaps badly—me, my other kids, my young nephews who lived with us? What kind of strength could I draw from it as I faced the seemingly inevitable institutionalization of my own son? It's not that Lennie from *Of Mice and Men* and Charlie from *Flowers for Algernon* no longer resonated for me. But my tears now felt cheap and manipulated. How neatly those characters' tragic fates plotted on the classic narrative arc; how bloodless their sacrifices! Suddenly it seemed as if the greatest indictment one could level against anything was this: *it's not real.*

But Ben was real, and how I responded to him mattered. At least, my husband, Andy, thought it did. He told me my silence in the music class represented a "moral failure." He didn't care how awkward it would have been to approach a total stranger, or how unlikely it was that she would take my word over that of her doctor, who obviously had never suggested a problem of this magnitude. Andy knew, as I did, about the importance of early intervention for children with autism. "You have a responsibility to the child," he said, simply.

My friends with autistic kids didn't agree. "Never again," Stacey announced, when I asked her if she had ever diagnosed someone else's child. "Nothing good has ever come from it." She reported that previous observations were met only with anger. One acquaintance never spoke to Stacey again—even after official confirmation that her daughter was on the severe end of the autistic spectrum. Another friend, Melanie, who held a leadership position in the Philadelphia chapter of Cure Autism Now (which later merged with Autism Speaks), admitted that she was reluctant to confront parents because "they don't want to hear it."

Genuinely conflicted over what I should have done, I started what would become my first published essay. I had an indirect connection to an editor at the relatively new parenting website Babble (since acquired by Disney), but I was hesitant: like virtually every other MFA graduate I knew, I turned my nose up at digital publishing—the platform, we all agreed, of the hoi polloi. I honestly would rather have had my work appear in a paper journal read by five people (four of them college librarians) than posted online. But the essay was finished, nonfiction wasn't really my field, and print journals took months to reply. It just seemed easier to send it to Babble, which accepted it immediately.

If few people read literary journals, absolutely none of them respond. So I wasn't at all prepared for the hundreds of comments I received. Many of them were from other parents of severely autistic children, who wished someone had suggested they pursue an evaluation earlier, but others were critical—even though, in the end, I never did tell the mother I thought her son was autistic. As I wrote in the essay, when I couldn't stop thinking about Ben two weeks later, I went back to his music class. His mother wasn't there; instead, Ben was under the care of a nanny who seemed to really care about him, bouncing him on her back to the beat, roughhousing with him in the way so many autistic kids tend to love. I made sure to sit next to her and chatted the way women in music class always do. As the teacher was wrapping up, I mentioned that Ben reminded me of my oldest son at that age. I didn't mention autism at all, just that Jonah was a late talker—an approach my sister recommended as being less frightening and confrontational. I asked the nanny to tell Ben's mother that, because of his obvious language delay, he qualified for free speech therapy from the county's Early Intervention Unit, and she said she would.

The hostility of some of the commenters made me wonder if they even read that far. Or perhaps their anger at the idea of diagnosing someone else's child was so great they considered me a bad person just for raising the possibility. Now, after dozens of online publishing experiences, I've come to understand that vitriol is part of the territory. I've been attacked simply for having five children and for daring to take those five children to a restaurant—never mind my more obviously controversial positions on the categorization, perception, and treatment of autism. But almost a decade later, I still hadn't satisfactorily answered the question that preoccupied me in those days after my essay was posted: What is so wrong with suggesting to another parent that her child may be autistic?

THE ARGUMENTS RAISED by my detractors basically fell into three main objections. Some commenters pointed out that because I'm not a doctor, I wasn't qualified to make such an assessment. But honestly, it's not that hard. Parents of children on the spectrum often joke about their "autism radar"—being able to swiftly identify the one autistic kid in a crowd, sometimes by something as seemingly insignificant as how he moves his fingers. But in Ben's case, my autism radar wasn't triggered by one small oddity. Autism has very particular social and behavioral symptoms, and the more severe the manifestation, the easier they are to spot. When a child exhibits delays in language and socialization, along with strange movements like covering his ears and repetitively touching his hands together, there's no doubt an evaluation is in order.

It's not just autism: living with any disorder makes you an expert. And every time I conjured analogous situations, I couldn't help but think the reactions would have been very different. If one mother approached another on a public playground, for example, and said, "Excuse me, I couldn't help noticing your son blinking and staring off into space . . . my daughter has absence seizures and they look very much like that, you might want to take him to a neurologist," I couldn't imagine any response besides, "I will, thank you so much for pointing that out." Or if a stranger gently remarked on an irregularly shaped mole because she had just been treated for melanoma, or a bull's-eye rash because hers had turned out to be Lyme disease, or a bluish, swollen calf because she had almost died from a blood clot, would anyone dismiss those concerns simply because they didn't come from an MD?

Other readers warned me to stay away from their "quirky kids." This rejection of the medicalization of neurological variance is a core tenet of the neurodiversity movement, which argues that autism isn't a disease but a different way of seeing the world. Just beginning to gain traction in 2007, neurodiversity baffled me from the beginning—which didn't stop it from producing some of the most influential figures in the broader disability rights movement, including the former Autistic Self Advocacy Network president Ari Ne'eman and the writer John Elder Robison. Neurodiversity just had no connection to our lived experience with autism. "Quirky" was charming, it was adorable—it was Zooey Deschanel walking a potbellied pig down the streets of Manhattan in her fuzzy slippers. It was not kids banging their heads against the wall, yelling all night, or shoving their favorite DVDs down the toilet.

This isn't to say that there aren't quirky autistic people—those who are mildly affected may be able to thrive in mainstream environments, yet betray their diagnoses through unusual obsessions with baseball statistics, 1950s show tunes, amphibians, and so on. But the crucial thing about "quirky" is that, by definition, it is firmly rooted in the functional realm. No one looks at an eleven-year-old in a pull-up diaper and a helmet who can't engage in reciprocal conversation but can recite *101 Dalmatians* in its entirety and observes, "That's one quirky kid."

The problem is, it's difficult to know at two whether a toddler will grow into that eleven-year-old or a quirky kid. I'm confident I speak for the overwhelming majority of parents of severely autistic children when I say that we all thought our kids would be quirky kids. We really believed it. We read the books about children who lost their diagnoses through special diets, supplements, and therapies. We saw other students make great progress with applied behavior analysis. We nurtured every splinter skill, clinging to the hope that our kids' precocious abilities to dispatch child-proof locks and navigate extraordinarily complex entertainment systems would evolve into problem-solving competencies sufficient for college, career, and ultimately, independent living.

Andy and I believed it for a long time. But that didn't stop us from exhausting our county's early intervention services, procuring speech and occupational therapy, and securing Jonah's admission to the best autism classroom in our school district. Andy has a favorite saying: "Trust in Allah, but tie your camel." The autism diagnosis is determined by clinical professionals and based on very strict criteria. I have never heard of a single parent who received that diagnosis and breezed out of the doctor's office, confident her quirky kid didn't need any labels or special services. Quirky is the best possible outcome of an autism diagnosis. It's typically not where it starts.

The final theme was also the most puzzling: "Mind your own business." Obviously, we all have countless inconsequential opinions about others we should keep to ourselves. But when it matters, we owe each other more than that. Who wouldn't pull a struggling swimmer out of the water, cry out to a person about to step into traffic, or call the police to report a burglar breaking into a home? Not everyone does, of course. In troubling cases including the 2012 rape of a high school student by football players in Steubenville, Ohio, and the 2017 drowning of a Florida disabled man, the failure of bystanders to even pick up the phone and call 911 precipitated national moral crises over so-called bad Samaritanism, which the Fordham law professor Peter J. O'Connor has called "the ugly side of human nature."[2] As of 2009, ten states had passed "duty to rescue" statutes.[3]

What about when a life isn't on the line? Perhaps we're no longer obligated, but I'm hard pressed to think of helpful, well-intentioned interventions that aren't appreciated. I have lowered my window to tell another driver his headlight was out, and flashed my own brights to warn of an upcoming speed trap. I've flicked a bee off a stranger's sleeve, volunteered to take a picture of tourists in front of Independence Hall, and offered a cough drop to a sick patron at the theater. I've helped an elderly woman load a heavy bag of cat food into her trunk and given up my seat on the train to a mother and her baby—and never, not once, was I met with a snarl: "Mind your own business! Maybe I like driving with just one headlight, did you ever think of that?"

"It's not the same," Keri said at the time. But why not? Is it because our protective instincts are automatically triggered once our kids are involved? I began to wonder what the response would have been if my essay had been about *disciplining* other people's children, rather than diagnosing them. I could imagine the same angry objections: "You're not an expert"; "Hands off my independent/assertive/spirited child"; and, of course, "Mind your own business." Then, in May 2016, I found out: the blogger Karen Alpert addressed this exact issue in her post "Dear Stranger Who

Disciplined my Kiddo at the Playground Today." Speaking directly to the mother who scolded Alpert's son for being too aggressive on the monkey bars, Alpert wrote, "I didn't get the chance to say this today, but THANK YOU. Because if my kid is acting like a douchenugget and I'm not around for whatever reason, you have my permission to tell him to knock that shit off." She went on to acknowledge, "yeah, I know there are probably a-holes out there who would be all pissy about some stranger getting mad at their kiddo, but not me."[4]

The post went viral; it was shared on Facebook almost three million times. Although a few of the five hundred-plus comments left on the original post did in fact get pissy, such as one reader who protested, "OMG! Nobody talks to my kid! You got a problem? Come to me! I won't have my child scarred for life because a stranger yells at them," the vast majority sided with Alpert— including someone who replied directly to the offended commenter, "Thank goodness people like you are few and far between." Overall, the responses reflected Alpert's final observation: "It takes a village. And these days our village might be a little bigger . . . and we don't even all know each other, but we can either choose to have a village or not. And I choose to have a village."

So do I. But I guess not too many people want to live in my village. When it comes to autism, the analogies fail, and the gratitude disappears. What I couldn't figure out, in the decade since my essay was published by Babble, is why.

A LOT CHANGED for me in those years. My kids grew up; I no longer had any toddlers or spent much time around them, so I never again ran into an undiagnosed autistic child. Maybe that was because autism awareness became so ubiquitous there just weren't any. Pediatricians began incorporating developmental assessments into wellness visits for babies as young as nine months. Today it's hard to imagine a child who, like Jonah, didn't point or follow one-step directions making it to his second birthday before raising any red flags.

Eventually, I gave up fiction almost entirely—writing it and even reading it. What I had always enjoyed about fiction were the fascinating questions raised by my favorite novels: What would it be like living in a postapocalyptic world (*The Stand*, by Stephen King)? How might terrorists and their hostages come to care about one another under an extended confinement (*Bel Canto*, by Ann Patchett)? What would happen if some fraction of the population just disappeared (*The Leftovers* by Tom Perrotta)? These authors explore possible answers, but certainly would never claim to have the only answer, or even the correct answer. What they would probably say, if asked (and as a former fiction writer, I feel like I can say this with confidence), is that there is no right answer. The point is just to ask questions that will make readers think. If they're still thinking months or even years later, score that as a win.

But there's nothing like having a disabled child to make you realize that there is, for most questions, a right answer. If we could run a Monte Carlo simulation for every decision we face—somehow access an infinite series of alternate universes in which we could pick each and every option and see what happens next—we would find out that, even if the choices seemed close or even interchangeable up front, that one in fact did lead to the best possible outcome. That's not to say there wouldn't be many other good, even great, results for many people making many different kinds of decisions. My oldest daughter, Erika, for example, has wanted to be a veterinarian since she could pronounce the word. Perhaps an experiment like the one I just described would prove that she actually would be happiest if she followed that dream. But I have no doubt that if she changed her mind at some point and became a geneticist or a biology teacher or a patent attorney, she would also be very happy. I imagine her at this point in her life as standing at the center of a giant wheel, the countless spokes representing all the diverse paths she could choose: different fields of study, jobs, cities. And I don't worry about her future, because I know she doesn't really have any bad options.

Jonah's life I imagine very differently: a narrow road with a series of forks, like the one faced by Belle's father in the animated movie *Beauty and the Beast*, where one side leads to certain glory at the science fair and the other to a terrifying wolf attack and, ultimately, a lifetime of imprisonment in the Beast's dungeon.[5] I don't know one other parent of a severely autistic child who doesn't feel this unbearable pressure, the need to make the right decision at each and every juncture: the right school, the right medication, the right therapy that will maximize our kids' potential, autonomy, and quality of life. Only these choices aren't clearly marked, as Maurice's were, by sunny skies and chirping birds on one hand and ominous shadows and creeping fog on the other. Instead, we must sort through a deluge of anecdotal evidence, internet reports, inconclusive studies, and often contradictory medical opinions. Is it any wonder that so many of us spent the years immediately following our children's diagnoses in a frenzy of alternative treatments and expensive therapists? We knew how illogical it was, that diets or vitamins or deep pressure or modulated sounds or hyperoxygenated air could alleviate significant neurological deficits. But so many roads led to the dungeon: the school expulsion, the abusive group home, the locked ward. How could we live with ourselves if we passed up the one thing that might have worked?

I, like many parents, emerged from this period with a profound respect for facts. Not much more is certain about autism causes, treatment, or prognoses now than when Jonah was a toddler. Researchers have validated the efficacy of applied behavior analysis and confirmed that two antipsychotics can reduce agitation associated with autism, but many kids fail to respond. Controlling the more devastating symptoms, such as aggression, self-injury, property destruction, pica, and elopement, is still often a heartbreaking process of trial and error. But my belief that Jonah would grow up to be a quirky kid has been replaced by an unwavering faith that science will eventually provide solutions to even the most vexing issues plaguing the autism community.

That conviction, I suspect, finally ended my lifelong love affair with fiction. Why read books that simply raised interesting questions, when instead I could read books that raised interesting questions—and then answered them? Most of what I picked up was at least peripherally concerned with neurology—such as *The Man Who Wasn't There*, by Anil Ananthaswamy, or Susannah Cahalan's memoir *Brain on Fire*. But, ultimately, it didn't matter whether the questions were related to autism or not. I loved learning about the techniques mastered by the USA Memory Champion Joshua Foer in *Moonwalking with Einstein* and the secrets of super-endurance athletes Christopher McDougall uncovered in *Born to Run*. For me, answers of any kind are inherently satisfying.

Occasionally, I've found, those answers illuminate different questions altogether—like why the idea of diagnosing someone else's child provokes so much anger. Economics professor Bryan Caplan introduced the concept of "rational irrationality" in his 2008 book *The Myth of the Rational Voter*. He argues, "Worldviews are more a mental security blanket than a serious effort to understand the world. . . . No wonder human beings shield their beliefs from criticism, and cling to them if counterevidence seeps through their defenses." No news here, but what Caplan concludes is that it is *rational* for us to act in this way when the cost is cheap, as it is in voting: "If one vote cannot change policy outcomes, the price of irrationality is zero."[6] The price of changing our worldview, however, and perhaps relinquishing the comfort and security it provides, can be quite steep.

Is there any worldview more cherished than that our babies have unlimited potential, that they will grow into autonomous adults, that they will surpass us in intelligence, character, popularity, and achievement? Nothing threatens that worldview more than an autism diagnosis. In its most severe manifestations, autism impairs every capacity we use to engage the world—understanding, communication, self-control, empathy—resulting in complete dependence. Other serious childhood disorders offer clear treatment protocols, hopeful prognoses, even cures. So Caplan's theory would predict that parents faced with the possibility that their children may have, for example, cancer or epilepsy would react more practically; as he notes, "People tailor their degree of rationality to the costs of error."[7] The potential cost of ignoring symptoms of these diseases is preventable death. Autism, however, is generally perceived as an irremediable, lifelong condition. While early intervention and other therapies can improve outcomes, most people untouched by the disorder don't know that. So clinging to their worldviews risks very little. There is no need to rush to the doctor on the say-so of one stranger in a music class: autistic children will still be autistic tomorrow.

It seems like an odd lesson that those of us who, like the Greek prophetess Cassandra, have certain kinds of truly impactful information should just keep quiet because no one will ever believe us. And that isn't Caplan's final takeaway. While it may be true that my belief in Ben's autism would have been met with hostility had I shared it with his mother, that doesn't mean it wouldn't have made a difference in his life. Caplan cites the findings of the researchers Colin Camerer and Robin Hogarth: "Useful cognitive capital probably builds up slowly, over days of mental fermentation or years of education."[8] In other words, Ben's mom might very well have rejected the possibility at first. But further thought, and perhaps additional comments about Ben's delays or unusual mannerisms from a grandparent or babysitter, might together have pushed through that initial resistance and caused her to seek out an evaluation sooner or, at the very least, to be more prepared for the recommendation when it inevitably came from her pediatrician. Perhaps my suggestion that she take advantage of the free speech therapy provided by the county served a similar function— I hope it did. Because I do believe we are all, in some ways, responsible for one another. If that connection were all fun and easy, it would be symbolized by a frat party, not a village. Instead it is our darkest moments, the expertise we never wanted, that most inform our answers—particularly to those dim, inchoate questions that check, or even defy, articulation.

4

The Next Time

One cold February night, a friend of mine and I took our combined eight kids out to dinner. Jonah was, naturally, very excited about the imminent arrival of his hamburger and french fries; he bounced in his seat, clapped his hands, and vocalized in a mishmash of squeals and catchphrases from his favorite *Sesame Street* videos. He wasn't exceedingly loud, but the oddness of his behavior had clearly caught the attention of an older gentleman at the one other table occupied at that early hour.

"Shhhhhhhh," he hissed from across the room.

Everyone at the table instantly froze—except, of course, for Jonah. "I'm sorry," I explained, rising from my seat and taking a few steps towards him so I wouldn't have to holler. "My son is autistic—"

"Oh. Sorry," he said.

"He's not trying to disturb you intentionally—"

"I heard you the first time," he snapped.

My face burned as I returned to my seat, his gratuitous nastiness instantly draining the joy from the evening. I spent the rest of the dinner constantly shushing Jonah, even though we had specifically decided to eat out at six o'clock on a Thursday night in a casual eatery precisely so we wouldn't have to hold any of the kids to impossible standards of behavior.

I suppose I should have been glad it ended there. Recently, another Pennsylvania family was kicked out of a Friendly's because their autistic five-year-old was crying; a Tennessee mother was also asked to leave a pizzeria because her autistic toddler was disturbing other customers.[1] Autistic kids have been escorted off airplanes, expelled from public gardens, and, ironically enough, ejected from *Finding Dory*, a children's movie commonly interpreted as a story about disability.[2] Each and every time the news reports incidents like these, online debates erupt between those who plead for empathy and inclusion, arguing that "every child even those children with Autism should be able to enjoy being out in the community!"[3] and those who berate parents for expecting others to accommodate their kids' disruptive behavior (such as one reader who commented on the *Dory* post, "Waaaaahhhh!! Another selfish mom whining that her special child did not get special treatment," or another who put it even more succinctly, "Grow up lady! Wait for the DVD").

That's certainly one option. I know plenty of families who simply don't take their autistic children out in the community, unless it's to special events catered to this population. And there are increasingly more of these to choose from: zoos, amusement parks, bowling alleys, roller skating rinks, movie theaters, and purveyors of just about any type of entertainment imaginable are setting aside time specifically for individuals with autism. These are fabulous programs that allow autistic kids to have fun and try new activities while taking the pressure off parents, who don't have to worry that their children are being too loud or just too weird— because I suspect it's often the strangeness of autistic behavior that disturbs people, not simply the volume. My four younger kids have done their share of enthusiastic joking and singing in restaurants and other public spaces, but no one has questioned the appropriateness of their presence as some have done after observing Jonah chant, "Mommy, Aunt Keri with a Daddy song" while wiggling his fingers in front of his face until he goes cross-eyed.

There's no question that separation makes things easier for everyone. After another older patron at the same establishment complained on a different night about Jonah watching his iTouch while waiting for his dinner, we permanently moved our group into a party room apart from the main dining room. I was finally able to relax—we didn't have to make Jonah stay in his seat, or constantly remind the seven other kids to use their "indoor voices." Philosophically, however, it bothered me: What were my children, and my friend's children, learning about the place of the disabled in the community? Would they grow up thinking it's perfectly natural for people like Jonah to literally be shunted into a back room?

SCHOLARS HAVE LONG argued against the depiction of the physically and intellectually disabled as "other," which the feminist theorist Susan Wendell defines as follows:

> When we make people "Other," we group them together as the objects of our experience instead of regarding them as subjects of experience with whom we might identify, and we see them primarily as symbolic of something else—usually, but not always, something we reject and fear and project onto them. To the non-disabled, people with disabilities . . . symbolize, among other things, imperfection, failure to control the body, and everyone's vulnerability to weakness, pain and death.[4]

Unfortunately, that in-group/out-group mentality is hard-wired in our species. Those early human ancestors who were genetically predisposed to form and maintain groups were much more reproductively successful in their extraordinarily perilous environment than those who tried to go it alone. As a result, according to Edward O. Wilson, the founder of the field of sociobiology (otherwise known today as evolutionary psychology), we've developed an "overpowering instinctual urge to belong to groups." Wilson adds, "We tend to think of our own group as superior, and we define our personal identities as members within them."[5]

Psychological research repeatedly confirms this bias, which appears at a very young age. A 2006 study by Meagan Patterson and Rebecca Bigler found that preschool students who were arbitrarily given red or blue T-shirts to wear for three weeks developed preferences for their own groups even when their teachers ignored the difference, making the categories meaningless.[6] This was hardly surprising to social psychologists; decades earlier, Henri Tajfel elicited intergroup discrimination by dividing teenage boys into groups based solely on whether they preferred abstract paintings by Paul Klee or Wassily Kandinsky, or whether they tended to over- or underestimate the number of dots flashed on a screen.[7] And, most famously, Philip Zimbardo was forced to abort his 1971 Stanford Prison Experiment after only six days because of the physical and emotional abuse suffered by subjects who had been randomly assigned the roles of "prisoners" at the hands of those given the roles of "guards."[8]

These studies document in-group/out-group behavior based on superficial or even chance distinctions. Imagine how much easier it is to draw the line at an obvious, critical difference like intellectual disability. Arguably, there is no more salient boundary; since the dawn of civilization, philosophers such as Plato and Aristotle have celebrated human rationality as the critical feature of our species—Plato supported the enslavement of non-Greeks with "unprivileged minds" and even endorsed the "exposure of all feeble children."[9] Later thinkers stopped short of explicitly endorsing infanticide and slavery, but in a way their conclusions were worse: In the late seventeenth century, John Locke defined the severely intellectually disabled right out of personhood with his definition of a "person" as "a thinking intelligent being that has reason and reflection and can consider itself as itself."[10]

Modern philosophers such as Peter Singer and Jeff McMahon have taken Locke's definition to its logical extreme, comparing the profoundly cognitively impaired to animals. Singer asks, "Why should there be any fundamental inequality of claims between a dog and a human imbecile?"[11] There shouldn't be, agrees McMahon: "It is difficult to identify any intrinsic difference between the severely retarded and animals with comparable psychological capacities that is relevant to the morality of killing them."[12] Although the two scholars insist their stated intent is not to demean the intellectually disabled but to raise the status of animals—both oppose eating meat—their protestations strike me as a bit disingenuous. Such comparisons inevitably lower the status of Jonah and his peers.

Singer and McMahon's dehumanizing language shouldn't be dismissed as mere metaphor or rhetoric. Studies examining abuse rates in the intellectually and developmentally disabled report a range of prevalence levels, from just over 60 percent to a staggering 90 percent.[13] A 2016 report from the *Chicago Tribune* uncovered cases of group home staff locking residents in their rooms, restraining them with duct tape, mocking their disabilities, and leaving them to sit in soiled clothing or sleep on dirty mattresses.[14] In New York, four direct care workers were charged with forcing residents to battle one another in "a developmentally disabled fight club" that evokes images of dog fighting.[15]

This is not to suggest that these abusive aides actually read the work of Singer or McMahon. But they obviously share a similar attitude toward the developmentally disabled. Philip Zimbardo, who never really recovered from the cruelty he witnessed in his own lab more than forty years ago, has spent the rest of his career studying how seemingly nice, normal people can do the terrible things his "guards" did to his "prisoners": insult them, deprive them of sleep, prod them with batons, force them to clean latrines with their bare hands, and sexually humiliate them. He places a good chunk of the blame on how easily and naturally dehumanization occurs once group lines have been drawn. "Dehumanization is the central construct in our understanding of 'man's inhumanity to man,'" Zimbardo writes. "[It] occurs whenever some human beings consider other human beings to be excluded from the moral order of being a human person."[16] Sound familiar? "Excluded from the moral order of being a person." That line could have been written by Singer or McMahon.

Disability rights organizations like Not Dead Yet and the Alliance Center for Independence have unsurprisingly protested Peter Singer's work in particular. But as important as it is to fight against the dehumanization of the disabled, we must be very careful how we throw that word around. Recently, some advocates have targeted the last group in the world one would expect to marginalize the intellectually and developmentally disabled: their parents. The writer Paul Solotaroff's 2016 essay about his autistic son Luke had been live on the *Rolling Stone* website less than twenty-four hours before the neurodiversity proponents Emily Willingham and Shannon Rosa posted blistering critiques, both specifically accusing Solotaroff of "dehumanizing" the disabled. What, exactly, did he do? According to Rosa, he "expos[ed] Luke's most vulnerable moments," a sentiment echoed almost verbatim by Willingham.[17]

This is undeniable. Solotaroff described the Clifford books his son still favored at the age of seventeen, his need for help bathing and toileting, his minimal language, the complete lack of safety awareness that made him a constant threat to dash into traffic. Solotaroff painted a very clear picture of a teenager whose severe deficits made him function more like "an ebullient toddler."[18]

But these details are only "dehumanizing" if such impairments are not part of the human experience (as, say, breathing underwater or laying eggs is not). Willingham points out that up to 25 percent of us will eventually become disabled; other writers, like Susan Wendell, argue the number is closer to 100 percent: "Unless we die suddenly, we are all disabled eventually."[19] Many of us may end up with support needs similar to Luke's—from traumatic brain injury, disease, or dementia. Do we then cease to be persons? At what point in our degeneration do we lose our status? I can't help but think of Lisa Genova's moving novel *Still Alice*, which traces the deterioration of a Harvard professor suffering from early-onset Alzheimer's. Planning to kill herself before her disease becomes too advanced, Alice programs her BlackBerry to ask her five questions each morning: "1. What month is it? 2. Where do you live? 3. Where is your office? 4. When is Anna's [her daughter's] birthday? 5. How many children do you have?" The message concludes, "If you have trouble answering any of these, go the file named 'Butterfly' on your computer and follow the instructions [to overdose on stashed pills] there immediately."[20]

The point is, we move in and out of rational states throughout the course of our lives—infancy, early childhood, accident, illness, psychosis, senescence—or even, depending who you ask, the course of our days: several scholars have pointed out that no one is rational while asleep, anesthetized, or intoxicated. Wonders the physician and ethicist John Wyatt, "Can something so fundamental as personhood be so fragile?"[21]

Increasingly, many feminist and disability theorists say no, rejecting reason as the necessary and sufficient condition for personhood. Eva Feder Kittay observes, "Nazi doctor murderers . . . employed rationality of a highly developed sort . . . yet the contributions of these capacities to sound moral agency were nil."[22] She proposes an alternative definition of "person," which would mean "having the capacity to be in certain relationships with other persons, to sustain contact with other persons, to shape one's own world and the world of others."[23] While this would greatly expand the category of persons, the Penn State professor Michael Bérubé, who has a son with Down syndrome, objects, "Any performance criterion—independence, rationality, capacity for mutual cooperation, even capacity for mutual recognition—will leave some mother's child behind."[24]

This is why human rights theories are so appealing. The sociologist Allison Carey notes,

> Philosophies of human rights seek to support all people, regardless of their abilities and backgrounds, in living lives that are meaningful and respectful of their humanity. They recognize that all people have needs and that these needs vary by person, by context, and over the life course, so that there is no clear division of people in need versus citizens. They also recognize our social obligation to create just and respectful societies rather than espouse pure individualism and meritocracy. Human-rights philosophies allow us to position people with disabilities, including people with significant disabilities, alongside other citizens as equal and valuable members, whereas liberalism and civic republicanism too often fail to do so.[25]

Admittedly, human-rights-based theories offer little to either the hypothetical Superchimp[26] (an enhanced chimpanzee with an intellect equivalent to that of an eleven-year-old child) or the advanced Martians featured in Jeff McMahon's attacks against such "speciesist" doctrines.[27] Neither do they benefit solely the severely intellectually disabled McMahon and Singer seek to exclude. Everyone gains when society grows more inclusive. From a purely quid pro quo perspective, don't we all hope to be gently guided home if we wander away one day in the throes of dementia? Wouldn't it be easier to face our futures if we knew that our neighbors would shovel a path in the snow for our wheelchairs, or that our fellow theater patrons would gracefully pretend our ventilators didn't disturb them? As Eva Feder Kittay points out, nothing less is at stake than the type of society we want to build: "Philosophers . . . have understated the critical role other capacities play in our moral life, capacities that we would want to encourage in the members of a moral community, such as giving care and responding appropriately to care, empathy, and fellow feeling; a sense of what is harmonious and loving; and a capacity for kindness and an appreciation for those who are kind."[28] Perhaps that is why, when the United Nations decided to codify its position on rights in 1948, it declined to define personhood or celebrate any particular qualifying traits and chose instead a human-rights-based paradigm. In a proclamation appropriately titled The Universal Declaration of Human Rights, the assembly declared, "Recognition of the inherent dignity and of the equal and inalienable rights of all members of the human family is the foundation of freedom, justice and peace in the world."[29]

DOES THIS MEAN I should have handled the scene in the restaurant differently? Perhaps I should have said instead, "I'm sorry, my son is . . . a fellow human and an equal member of our moral community?"

If only it were that easy. Anyone who has ever been married knows the last thing in the world you should do if you hope to change someone's mind is challenge him or her directly. That doesn't mean people can't be persuaded—if the billions of dollars spent on advertising every year tell us anything, it's that our beliefs are influenced all the time, generally at the subconscious level. Social psychologists have researched extensively the science of attitude change, including Philip Zimbardo, who, after seeing how easily social factors pushed his subjects to act on their darkest impulses, spent decades asking how we could harness the power of the environment for good. The question is, What can we borrow from this field to shift in-group/out-group boundaries— or, as evolutionary psychologists imagine them, "moral circles"— to include the intellectually and developmentally disabled? The Harvard professor Steven Pinker advises that in order to stop dehumanization and marginalization we need to "understand the psychology of the circle well enough to encourage people to put all of humanity inside it," and notes that this is not as idealistic and impossible as it might sound, as "the moral circle has been growing for millennia."[30] (Interestingly, Peter Singer has also adopted this idea—even taking it for the title of his book *The Expanding Circle*—to argue that "the moral circle should therefore be pushed out until it includes most animals."[31])

The first step in the persuasive process, Zimbardo states, is exposure. Uncoincidentally, this also happens to be one of the main reasons parents give on blogs and other platforms for why they take their autistic children out in public, despite the judgmental looks and comments elicited by their often odd, sometimes disruptive behavior. "It's good for the public to get used to seeing people with differences out and about," writes Lauren Casper for the disability website The Mighty. "It's good for us as a society to learn to live together in unity. . . . One of the ways we do that is by being together, in public, with all kinds of people of all kinds of abilities."[32] A. Stout for The Autism Site agrees: "The world needs to be exposed to children with autism. . . . Countless myths and stereotypes abound. . . . Allowing children with autism to interact with the public allows people to see the truth."[33]

And what is the truth? That our kids love going out, just like the rest of us do. They love eating hamburgers and french fries, trying all the free samples at Costco, and pressing their cheeks against the cold freezer doors—at least, Jonah does. And I have to think it's that unselfconscious, contagious joy that explains why employees at all Jonah's favorite haunts inevitably ask for him whenever Andy or I show up alone. Maybe they never saw a kid before who jumped up and down and clapped while reciting fragments of *Sesame Street* videos, or dropped suddenly to the ground to press his hands against the smooth concrete floor, or tried to wedge himself behind cases of soda or laundry detergent. But after watching Jonah every week, I imagine those behaviors became less and less distracting, until staff members were touched when they looked at him, not by what was strange, but by what wasn't: the way he affectionately loops his arm through his father's; his constant requests for "more" of everything, "*please*"; his obvious appreciation for places that most people find too mundane to get excited about. I know I'm being speculative, but I really can't think of another reason. Those cashiers and waitresses and security guards never ask about any of our other kids.

People who routinely encounter individuals like Jonah in the community—running the same errands, enjoying the same activities, and yes, even struggling with things that come easily for others—may be more likely to engage with them. Zimbardo recommends a strategy called the "foot-in-the-door" technique[34] to shift attitudes: start small. Last spring, for example, I took Jonah to an indoor water park by myself. I was a bit apprehensive how

I would manage it—unlike amusement park rides, which Jonah and I board and disembark together (and, not irrelevantly, are strapped in for the duration), water slides often require us to go sequentially. That meant I would either have to send Jonah down first, and hope he would promptly exit the pool and wait for me (unlikely), or I would have to go first myself and pray that Jonah's desire to go down the slide was stronger than the temptation to take advantage of the momentary lack of supervision and sneak back down the stairs to steal a treat from the snack bar. My plan to ask the lifeguard stationed at the top of the slides for help was abandoned as soon as I saw how many slides he had to monitor.

Ultimately, I just asked the person behind me in line to keep an eye on Jonah and make sure he didn't go down the slide until it was safe. Nobody ever said no. And we had a great time: Jonah listened and followed directions, and because he did, not only was he able to stay at the park as long as he wanted but I promised him we could go back again soon.

What about the strangers I enlisted? The foot-in-the-door technique predicts that, having done this small thing for us, they would be more likely to make a more involved commitment in the future. Perhaps next time they see a family like ours in a supermarket or fast-food restaurant they might offer to let them step in front of the line. (I believe there's no empathetic gesture that beats this one, in terms of pure value. It costs so little, but often makes a tremendous difference for that family, who may have been forced to leave—without their lunch, or their groceries—because of their child's increasing agitation.) Perhaps they will encourage their own children to approach kids like Jonah on the playground, invite group home residents in their neighborhood for a dip in their swimming pool, or donate to an autism nonprofit.

And don't forget about the contributions of other branches of psychology to the understanding of persuasion. Behaviorism emphasizes the importance of reinforcement; we do what we've been rewarded for doing in the past. So every happy shriek from Jonah, every expression of appreciation from me, every successful trip down the water slide facilitated by my recruits increases the likelihood of further engagement—and nudges that moral circle just a bit more open.

WHICH BRINGS ME, naturally, to porn.

Not real porn, but "inspiration porn"—the label that's recently been attached to viral videos or news accounts featuring a nondisabled person doing something nice for a disabled person. Recent examples include the elaborate "promposal" staged by the Florida cheerleader Mika Bartosik for her autistic classmate Jonathan Ramilo, featuring a giant cookie with "Will you go to the prom with me?" written on it, as well as the sacrifice by high school wrestler Devin Schuko of his perfect season to his opponent, Andy Howland, who has Down syndrome.[35] Disability rights proponents routinely denounce these stories; autistic self-advocate Kit Mead argues, echoing Susan Wendell, that inspiration porn portrays people with disabilities as "other—less than human, or a lower level of human. Because we are other, acts of kindness toward us seem newsworthy."[36]

But I think Mead is missing the point. Acts of kindness between strangers are newsworthy, period—particularly if they cross assumed in-group/out-group boundaries. Many similarly inspiring stories have swept the internet that have nothing to do with disability, such as an Alabama college student who mowed the lawns of the elderly in his neighborhood for free; an African American young man from New York who brought Starbucks treats to white police officers; and an employee of a Georgia Wal-Mart who literally gave the shoes off his feet to a homeless man.[37] I was even moved reading about the thousands of dollars North Carolina democrats raised to reopen a Republican headquarters that was firebombed in 2016.[38] I really believe most people are responding to the human connection portrayed in these stories when they click and share them, not the objectification of the disabled . . . and the elderly . . . and police officers . . . and Republicans?

The activist David Perry contends, "There's nothing real about these stories"—at least, the ones involving the disabled.[39] I'm not sure how anyone could watch Jonathan Ramilo carom around his classroom with joy and doubt the authenticity of that moment. I'm assuming Perry is referring to Mika and her unknown motivations. Although she appears sweet and enthusiastic, she might just have asked Jonathan to the prom to cultivate an experience worthy of a college admissions essay, or perhaps in hopes of getting exactly the attention and commendation she received.

Philip Zimbardo contends that Mika's original reasons don't really matter. "Beliefs follow behavior," he writes. "Get people to perform good actions, and they will generate the necessary underlying principles to justify them. Talmudic scholars are supposed to have preached not to require that people believe before they pray, only to do what is needed to get them to begin to pray; then they will come to believe in what and to whom they are praying."[40] He attributes this shift to the human need to resolve cognitive dissonance, or for "internal consistency between different cognitions in the mind of a person."[41] It would be very uncomfortable for Mika, for example, to believe that the intellectually disabled are subhuman while also knowing that she asked a person with intellectual disabilities to the prom. She can't very well pretend that the promposal never happened—over two hundred thousand people watched it on

YouTube. Notes Zimbardo and Lieppe, "When behavior cannot be changed or revoked, one or more of the beliefs or attitudes with which is it is inconsistent might be changed . . . in the service of seeing . . . current or past behavior as consistent, reasonable, and justified."[42] Ultimately, Mika's only option to resolve her dissonance would be to adopt a more inclusive attitude toward the disabled.

But that's not why I love inspiration porn—honestly, I believe the nondisabled actors in these stories are sincere. It's because of the potential impact on everyone else. These videos allow those who may have never met a person with an intellectual or developmental disability to gain much needed experience—indirect, no doubt, but perhaps enough to challenge stereotypes and prejudices. And the positive feedback very likely inspires others to act similarly (after all, it's called *inspiration* porn for a reason). Accumulating kindnesses will hopefully create a new group norm to which others will naturally conform—resulting in the embrace of Jonathan, Andy Howland, Jonah and all their intellectually disabled peers into the community's moral circle.

What might that look like? Welcoming the intellectually disabled into our public spaces would be an important part. Expecting individuals like Jonah to just stay home is completely incompatible with a just and inclusive society. Not all spaces, at all times: sharing only works if everyone is respectful and considerate. As the bioethicist Allen Buchanan notes, "Honoring the commitment to inclusiveness may require a mutual sacrifice of legitimate interests."[43] So I'm not going to take Jonah to opening night of the next *Star Wars* installment, or to a fancy French café on Valentine's Day. But I might take him to a noon showing of a movie that's been out for weeks. And I will definitely take him to family-friendly restaurants where it's unreasonable to expect much ambience, such as the one where we were scolded, or maybe the one featured in a

2012 segment of ABC's show *What Would You Do?* In this hidden-camera video, actors portraying a severely autistic teen and his family were universally supported against a single diner (also an actor) who was outraged by the boy's disruptive behavior. What had me sobbing in front of my computer was that even when the actor playing the autistic teen actually snatched french fries off the man's plate—something Jonah has tried to do, many times—the other patrons rallied behind the family, comforted the parents, and applauded when the man stormed out.

I've never allowed myself to hope for that much acceptance, but maybe I should. Many months after I first saw this video, I discovered that Andy's cousin Oliver Miede, in a staggering coincidence, had actually produced this segment. When I told him how much I loved it, he admitted how surprised he had been at the customers' unanimous reaction, even when they reenacted the scenario later in the day, with a different group of diners. "We didn't realize it when we scheduled the shoot, but that day school was closed, and many of the people in that restaurant were teachers," he said. "I wonder if that had anything to do with it?"

How could it be otherwise? Of course there are disinterested or even hostile teachers, but in general this is a service profession chosen by those who care about students and who become deeply invested in their progress. They have regular contact with children with intellectual and developmental disabilities, if not in their classrooms, then in their schools. I can't think of a profession whose members would be less likely to condemn kids like Jonah to the out-group. Maybe this is what an expanded moral circle looks like: strangers rallying to support the vulnerable, to comfort the persecuted, to accept the unacceptable.

Or maybe that's too much to ask. But I know we can do better than "I heard you the first time."

5

Just Say Yes

I pulled the amber bottle from its packaging and laid it across the palm of my hand. "PHARMA CBD ORAL SPRAY," stated the invoice. "PEPPERMINT." This product, according to a story that had popped up in my Facebook feed almost every time I recently opened it, had allegedly caused a nine-year-old autistic Puerto Rican boy to utter his first words.

I know better than to believe everything I read on the internet. But it wasn't just Kalel Santiago's breakthrough. I doubt there are many families caring for kids on the moderate-to-severe end of the spectrum who aren't aware of the notable benefits that have been reported from marijuana—in increasing engagement and communication, resolving aggressive and self-injurious behaviors, and controlling seizures. For many of us, the treatment remains tantalizingly unavailable, unless we're prepared to break the law. Instead we follow the very public stories of advocates whose sons have been prescribed cannabis legally—like Marie Myung-Ok Lee of Rhode Island, who published a four-part series on *Slate* about why she decided to give her nine-year-old marijuana, or the California mom Mieko Hester-Perez, who credits it with saving the life of her ten-year-old son.

While hemp oil is not derived from marijuana, it does contain CBD, one of its active ingredients. I had begun to wonder whether CBD might help Jonah with the myoclonic seizures he had been experiencing with increasing frequency—conscious events that at times resembled mild twitching but could escalate into a cluster of jerks and contractions that dropped him to the floor. I desperately wanted to avoid adding another medication to his regimen. The antiseizure drugs he had been prescribed as a young child to control his mood had terrible side effects—most notably a rapid weight gain that made him clinically obese within three months.

Even as I sprayed the CBD oil into Jonah's mouth, fantasizing about ultimately replacing all his other medical interventions with three minty spritzes, it seemed impossible to believe that a treatment I could buy online was powerful enough to stop seizures, calm aggression, and make the nonverbal speak. I couldn't help thinking about the *Simpsons* episode in which Homer finds out that bacon, ham, and pork chops all come from the pig. "Yeah, right, Lisa," he says in disbelief. "A wonderful, *magical* animal."[1] If CBD had half the effects attributed to it, I thought, watching Jonah for any immediate and unspecified reaction, it would in fact be nothing less than magical.

JENNIFER ABBANAT, A fellow member of a Facebook group for parents of kids with severe autism, has been treating her now fourteen-year-old son with various cannabis products for the past two years. Ty has autism and ADHD and suffered for most of his life from violent episodes in which he attacked his parents, punching and kicking them. "I have scars up and down my arms from all the pinches and scratches," Jennifer told me, when I asked if I could speak to her further about the massive improvements she had described in her posts. Her two daughters had a safety plan for when their brother raged. "They knew to go into my oldest daughter's room and lock the door," she said. "Ty didn't go after them directly, but once he started throwing things, anyone could get hit."

The family was tremendously isolated. Leaving the house was extraordinarily difficult for Ty because his sensory processing disorder often left him overwhelmed and anxious, provoking more meltdowns. "I couldn't drive the quarter of a mile to pick up my daughter at school without pulling over twice," Jennifer said.[2] Ty would take off his shoes and hurl them at her as she drove, or throw anything else he could find. Even if she successfully removed any potential missiles before leaving the house, Ty's compulsion to elope made him a threat at any moment to dash from the car.

His behaviors were dangerous for another reason: shortly after he was born, Ty was diagnosed with bowel disease that necessitated a cecostomy—the installation of a port through which fluids were introduced to flush his bowels—when he was four years old. Every night, his parents had to irrigate his bowels, a process that required him to sit on the toilet for an hour. If he didn't cooperate, he was at risk for impaction, which could require surgery, or even worse, a potentially fatal perforation.

"Twenty-fifteen was our summer of crisis," Jennifer told me. Ty had to be hospitalized for a surgical disimpaction; then he aspirated his gastric juices and developed pneumonia. "When he came home, he just really deteriorated," she said. "He couldn't sit still, every tiny thing threw him into a rage. That was the first time we ever had to call the police to come help." But the police couldn't offer much help—nobody could. Ty was turned away from the local pediatric psychiatric unit with no recommendations or referrals. "It turns out there's not a place on the West Coast that can take a kid with his medical *and* behavioral issues," Jennifer explained. "We felt very lost and hopeless, without any options."

That was when Jennifer and her husband decided to try marijuana, which she had been researching online for the past few years. Although Ty's psychiatrist was skeptical, she agreed to write a prescription for him because there was simply nothing left to try.

It was not an easy journey. Although in California, where Jennifer lives, medical marijuana is legal, she still had no professional guidance, no well-established protocol to follow. She went through several different strains and products—including Charlotte's Web CBD and another strain with equal amounts of CBD and THC—before trying THC oil. "This past year was amazing," Jennifer told me. "We've been able to replace all the psychotropics Ty was on—Abilify, Clonidine, and Valium—with two drops of a pure indica THC oil every five days. He is so much happier now. He's calm enough to sit for hours and read, or play with Legos, or even go for short rides in the car without incident. He still gets agitated sometimes, but I haven't been hit in well over seven months. Now, the worst thing he does is go out to the back deck and yell." She laughed. "Honestly, we're happy he's using his words."

Jennifer saw other positive effects in Ty she hadn't expected. "Ty was never able to sleep on his own," she told me. "For the past ten years, my husband has been sleeping with him. But just two months ago, Ty said he wanted to try sleeping like a big boy and now he is sleeping in his own bed without dad." Ty's sensory issues also resolved enough for the family to go camping with Jennifer's siblings and their kids—something he was never able to tolerate. Perhaps most significantly, Ty's bowel disease improved. "He's started to have his own bowel movements for the first time in his life," Jennifer reported. "And it's been more than two years since he's needed a surgical disimpaction—something he used to need every six months or so." In short? "THC has been a miracle."

But Jennifer, Marie Myung-Ok Lee, and Mieko Hester-Perez, as compelling as their stories are, don't count as real evidence, at least not to doctors and politicians. Science refers to such reports as "anecdotal," which always strikes me as hopelessly dismissive. Anecdotes are trifles, humorous snippets about colleagues or neighbors, not detailed accounts of transformative experiences like those experienced by these families. And I get it. I've tried enough therapies—diet, vitamins, hyperbaric oxygen treatment, brushing—to make me skeptical of any treatment that doesn't have an impeccable pedigree of double-blind, placebo-controlled studies supporting it.

But what if the reason why there are so few studies isn't lack of safety or efficacy but because the government has put up too many obstacles? Since the Controlled Substances Act was passed in 1970, access to marijuana—even for researchers—has been highly regulated. It is considered a Schedule I substance, which puts it in the company of heroin, LSD, ecstasy, and other drugs that have "no currently accepted medical use in treatment in the United States," according to the statute.[3]

But marijuana has been used medically for three thousand years, to treat conditions including insomnia, nausea, pain, seizures, and countless others. In fact, the Food and Drug Administration (FDA) has—paradoxically, given its Schedule I classification—approved certain medical marijuana studies, but the regulatory hurdles don't end there. Rick Doblin, executive director of the Multidisciplinary Association for Psychedelic Studies (MAPS) has been fighting with the National Institute on Drug Abuse (NIDA) and the Drug Enforcement Agency (DEA) for years to gain access to marijuana he needs to pursue projects already approved by the FDA. "We had one study looking at AIDS wasting and the other on migraines that were killed because NIDA refused to sell us the

marijuana," he told me. And Doblin's not allowed to get it anywhere else, even in states in which it's completely legal. All marijuana research is required by law to use cannabis grown by NIDA
at the University of Mississippi. "Now we have another study on
PTSD in vets that was approved by the FDA about four years ago
and NIDA still can't say when they'll be able to get us the strains
we need or how much they will cost. We could get them right now
in Colorado or California or other states but the DEA refuses to
authorize any other growers."[4] This monopoly, Doblin points out,
has had a chilling effect on research. Few scientists can afford to
spend five years trying to get a study off the ground.

A relatively recent change did streamline the process to some
extent. In June 2015, the Department of Health and Human Services announced that marijuana studies no longer need to be approved by the US Public Health Service—an additional layer of
bureaucracy that had delayed research by an average of one year.
But many experts in this field believe that much-needed studies
into marijuana's medical efficacy won't begin in earnest until the
classification is changed. "As long as marijuana continues to live
in that category [Schedule I], it's going to be . . . very difficult for
researchers to do studies that can help us figure out whether and
how it works," David Casarett, MD, argues in his book *Stoned:
A Doctor's Case for Medical Marijuana*. And after conducting dozens of interviews and extensively reviewing the literature, Casarett
concludes this shift is overdue: "There's enough evidence to justify
reclassifying the cannabinoids in marijuana as Schedule II drugs,
which include morphine and oxycodone. These are commonly
prescribed but are regulated." Although preliminary evidence is
strongest for marijuana's therapeutic effect on nausea and certain
types of pain, Casarett is intrigued by its potential benefits for
those suffering from Parkinson's disease, anxiety, dementia, even

cancer. Changing the classification "will make it easier to do randomized controlled trials," he writes.[5]

OF COURSE, MARIJUANA has been extensively researched—a keyword search in the search engine PubMed, which accesses a database of biomedical research maintained by the National Institutes of Health,[6] results in over twenty thousand hits—but the vast majority of studies have focused on the deleterious effects of recreational use. Contextualized by a drug war that has resulted in the arrest of over twenty million people for marijuana-related offenses, many of these reports have terrified parents with their findings that marijuana may make their children stupid and psychotic.

Concerns about effects on IQ, however, seem to be unsubstantiated. Although a 2012 study out of Duke University caused an international panic by confirming a "neurotoxic effect of cannabis on the adolescent brain," the *Washington Post* later reported on subsequent papers refuting that conclusion.[7] A much larger study by scientists from University College London, for example, found that marijuana had no effect on IQ "when confounding factors—alcohol use, cigarette use, maternal education, and others—were taken into account."[8]

This sloppy muddling of correlation and causation plagues much marijuana research, according to the Harvard professor emeritus and staunch cannabis advocate Lester Grinspoon, MD. "The most common finding is that marijuana makes kids lazy, or slothful. But that's nonsense,"[9] he told me. A much more likely explanation for this relationship, he suggests, is that disengaged, disaffected teens are more likely to use marijuana . . . as well as other mind-altering, illegal substances. This logic is supported by the British study, which did find one factor that was "strongly correlated" with loss of IQ: alcohol use, leading experts to posit what Grinspoon has known since he began studying marijuana in the 1960s—that our nation's myopic focus on marijuana use has obscured the dangers of other, more dangerous, adolescent behaviors.

Concerns about psychosis, however, are less easily dismissed. John Williams, MD, a child psychiatrist and past president of the Academy of Cognitive Therapy, has treated over two thousand patients of all ages for marijuana use. "The area which for me is of greatest concern is the apparent connection between THC and the development and worsening of psychotic illnesses," he said. Teens with a family history of bipolar disorder are most at risk. Williams has seen many who "developed hallucinations and delusions that resolved in many cases once marijuana use stopped," he told me. "But in some cases the effect has been permanent."[10]

Kevin M. Gray, MD, professor and director of child and adolescent psychiatry and professor of addiction sciences in the Department of Psychiatry and Behavioral Sciences at the Medical University of South Carolina, warns that "a number of psychiatric disorders are worsened with marijuana use, including psychotic disorders and mood disorders. I haven't seen any studies that show that marijuana can improve long-term outcomes in any psychiatric disorder. If there's any directionality, it's towards worsening."[11]

David Casarett agrees that studies connecting marijuana use to schizophrenia, another psychotic disorder, are concerning, but cautions, "There may be other causes . . . that might explain (and erase) what at first appears to be a clear case of cause and effect. In addition, other studies have found that marijuana use doesn't increase the risk of schizophrenia as much as a family history or a history of childhood abuse do."[12]

But, as Williams points out, autistic kids may share this genetic vulnerability. "There's a high comorbidity between bipolar disorder and autism," he said—in fact, Jonah was diagnosed with bipolar disorder in 2008. "And genetic studies show that bipolar 1 and schizophrenia tend to co-localize in families, so they probably represent genetically similar conditions."[13] All this might mean that autistic kids may be more likely to experience psychotic side effects than their neurotypical peers. Other factors, however, suggest they may be less likely; one 2013 study found altered endocannabinoid functioning in mouse models of autism, which means it may not be possible to predict how autistic brains will respond to marijuana based on research on neurotypical brains.[14]

The side effects of antipsychotics—the traditional treatment for aggressive and self-injurious behaviors in autistic kids—have, however, been well established. Accurate statistics are hard to come by, because reporting isn't mandatory, but between 2000 and 2006 over seventy children died from reactions to antipsychotics.[15] Thousands more suffered severe adverse reactions, including metabolic disorders, neuroleptic malignant syndrome, glaucoma, and potentially permanent muscular cramping. Weight gain is so ubiquitous that up to a third of kids became overweight or obese, some as quickly as eleven weeks after starting antipsychotics, according to one 2009 study.[16] And these are all relatively short-term side effects. As the FDA freely admits, long-term effects have never been tested. Yet it's completely legal for psychiatrists to prescribe antipsychotics to children, while medical marijuana is illegal for patients of all ages in more than a third of the states. Kevin Gray maintains that, given the current state of research, that's how it should be. "You seem to be very dismissive about what marijuana can do," he scolded me gently. "In terms of comparing risks to antipsychotics, that's a complicated comparison: very different effects, but very concerning with both. At least there's evidence that antipsychotics work."[17]

STILL FRUSTRATED WITH what I interpreted as complacency in the child psychiatrists I spoke with, I decided to consult a higher authority: Jonathan Moreno, a professor of bioethics at the University of Pennsylvania. For me, this issue isn't about side effects or efficacy studies, but an even more fundamental question: Who decides what treatments are available for our kids—the government, or parents and doctors? And even if we all agree that government oversight is necessary in general, don't the extreme crises many families are facing mandate a different set of rules? These ethical questions, I realize, don't necessarily fall under the purview of child psychiatry. Perhaps my problem is that I've been consulting the wrong kind of expert.

As it turns out, I leave Moreno's office disappointed. Although he is very supportive of Rick Doblin's work with MAPS, as well as a believer in decriminalization, his position is ultimately the same as that of Kevin Gray and John Williams: "I still want to see the studies done," he tells me. "I think it would be irresponsible not to start with studies." He advises against undermining the FDA process, which he argues "both protects people from fraud, and makes it more likely they get effective treatments rather than taking peach pits to alleviate their suffering. It took a long time and a lot of pain to get to where we are with drug approval. I understand that it takes a long time, and there are a lot of barriers—but, just like with democracy, the alternative is worse."[18]

To me this seems unnecessarily conservative, especially since Moreno acknowledges the lack of long-term studies of standard psychopharmacological treatments for dangerous behaviors. "This whole generation of kids is in a long-term experiment, spending forty to fifty years on Adderall and Zoloft. We have no idea what harm we may be doing," he said.

Given those unknown risks—combined with the well-established risks of untreated or unsuccessfully treated aggressive and self-injurious rages, during which autistic individuals have blinded and disfigured themselves, sustained irreversible brain damage, and significantly hurt or even killed their caregivers—isn't the government ethically obligated to lift the obstacles currently preventing the marijuana research everyone wants to see?

Moreno isn't willing to commit to that. But he does say, "If you could show marijuana was beneficial, the government would be ethically obligated to figure out a way of getting it to patients." So we're back to that vicious cycle: the government justifies its regulation of marijuana studies by pointing to the lack of randomized, placebo-controlled trials, but those studies can't be done until regulations are lifted.

And in the meantime, are parents like me supposed to just wait? Isn't our primary responsibility to find the best treatment for our children's extraordinarily debilitating condition?

Moreno agrees that, according to the ethical principle of autonomy, "Involved parents who love their kids are the best people to make health care decisions for them." However, he doesn't seem particularly troubled by the broad range of state laws that means some parents have to break the law in order to choose what may very well be the best treatment for their children, while others, like Jennifer, don't. Isn't this uneven accessibility troubling, if not, technically, unethical?

"There's all kinds of inequalities of access; that's a political philosophy question," Moreno says—which sounds like splitting hairs to me. "There's a lot of injustice in the world."

OH, WE KNOW about injustice, the parents of kids with severe developmental and intellectual disabilities. Haven't we been steeped in it from day one? It's *not fair* that our beautiful, blameless children have profound impairments that so greatly restrict their options. It's *not fair* that they will never live independently, never mind achieve any of the goals parents of neurotypical kids take for granted: college, career, marriage, parenthood. And because so much of our children's lots seems so unfair, it stings that much more when the government takes so little interest in a treatment with as much apparent potential as marijuana, which may be able to control those dangerous behaviors that so directly compromise our kids'—and our entire families'—quality of life. These aggressive and self-injurious behaviors, more than any other factor, including severity of disability, most directly predict physical and chemical restraint, expulsion from schools, day programs, and other services, and institutionalization. If Lester Grinspoon is right in his prediction that marijuana "will be *the* medicine used for these kids in the future,"[19] then there will be countless parents who will never forgive the government for failing to act sooner, for keeping from their children the medicine that might have allowed them to live safe and happy lives despite their significant challenges.

We are still far away from understanding whether marijuana can actually control dangerous behaviors in autism and, if so, how best to maximize those therapeutic benefits. Even parents with legal access to this treatment suffer from the complete dearth of knowledge about appropriate strains, preparation, and dosing. Karen Echols's autistic son, Alex, became the face of this debate after the media reported the dramatic reduction in self-injury he experienced immediately following his first exposure to a specific type of cannabis oil. "Before that, Alex needed to be wrapped in blankets almost all the time to keep him from head-banging and biting his arms from his hand to his shoulder," she told me. "But after we gave him the oil, we were able to unwrap him, and he could use his hands for exploring. We thought it was our miracle."[20]

However, the Echolses were unable to get consistent, stable results from marijuana. "We ran out of that particular oil," Karen said. "Even when we found a grower who had the strain we needed, we had to figure out how to turn the raw plant into an actual medicine. It was complete guesswork on our part. We tried glycerin tinctures, and cannabutter—sometimes they worked well, other times they didn't. It was hard to know if we were getting the concentration and the dosing right. We never saw a response as good as we did with the original oil." Ultimately, the family had to send Alex across the country for a six-month hospitalization. "We hope to try again when he hopefully moves closer to us," Karen added. "It was the best success we ever had."

This was a story I heard over and over again: marijuana worked, but then it didn't. Another Facebook friend, Tara, couldn't stop raving about the improvement in her twenty-three-year-old son, Jordan, when I first began researching this issue in 2014. "I was being attacked every day," she told me at the time. "I've blacked out after being hit in the head. I haven't been strong enough to manage him for a long time, so my strategy was to run and hide. Jordan broke his foot trying to break the door down to come after me." But Jordan's reaction to marijuana was immediate: "The second we put him on it, his mood improved, and his aggressions dropped from multiple times a day to once every week or ten days." Tara used the same word Jennifer did, telling me, "Marijuana is definitely a miracle cure for us when it comes to autism and aggression."[21]

But when I followed up with her in 2017, Tara was looking for an inpatient facility to treat Jordan's vicious rages, which frequently left her covered in ugly purple bruises. "After about eight months, the marijuana began to trigger intense OCD, which disintegrated into horrible violence," she told me. "We tried a large variety of strains, doses, and ways of ingesting from tinctures and edibles to pure raw plant material—we even had him puff a joint!—but we just couldn't repeat that great response we got at the beginning."[22]

David Casarett addresses this "common criticism of medical marijuana" in *Stoned*. "When the THC and CBD content of marijuana varies between buds, some people may not be getting an adequate dose. . . . That variability, it seems to me, makes it very difficult to call marijuana a 'medicine' in the same way that, say, penicillin is a medicine."[23] He predicts that, in the future, "there will be a lot of interest in testing synthetic cannabinoids."[24] Standardization can also be created in a lab, such as that of the British pharmaceutical company that designed Sativex, a drug that contains fixed doses of THC and CBD and is not yet available in the United States.

But Lester Grinspoon isn't convinced that either extracting THC and CBD or synthesizing them artificially will duplicate the medicinal effects of the whole plant. Besides these well-known components, marijuana contains over one hundred other cannabinoids and one hundred different molecules called terpenes, which, besides giving cannabis its distinctive odor, have their own therapeutic benefits. "Terpenes are essential for some reason," Grinspoon told me. "CBD is now synthesized separately, but it doesn't do anything. You can add a little THC and it still won't do anything, it has to have some terpenes in it to get what is known as the 'ensemble effect.'" Still, he remains optimistic: "We'll learn more about it," he said. "We were ignorant about CBD for years."[25]

Now, anyone with even a passing interest in medical marijuana is familiar with the different roles played by its major cannabinoids and the implications for the treatment of neurological symptoms.

While THC—the psychoactive ingredient in cannabis—relieves pain and nausea, CBD has anticonvulsant, antidepressant, and antipsychotic properties. In a case that made national headlines, a high-CBD, low-THC strain of marijuana brought relief to a five-year-old girl named Charlotte Figi with Dravet syndrome who was suffering three hundred grand mal seizures a week that had left her unable to talk, walk, or feed herself. After starting treatment with Charlotte's Web, the strain that was subsequently named after her, Charlotte's seizure frequency dropped to two or three times a *month*. Her amazing recovery was enough to change Sanjay Gupta's position on medical marijuana, as he reported in his 2013 CNN documentary, *Weed*.

Lester Grinspoon predicts that a strain with a high CBD to THC ratio "will become the workhorse" for treating autistic children with dangerous behaviors as well, because such variants "help the destructive symptoms without psychoactive effects." He added, "If I had an autistic kid, I would have a bunch of that available."[26]

But not everyone has a bunch of that available. Those who procure marijuana illegally almost certainly end up with strains that are high in THC and low in CBD, since recreational users aim to get as high as possible. In fact, most of the eight hundred strains that have been identified are high in THC for that reason, so even parents buying marijuana legally, through dispensaries, may not have access to the highest CBD options.

This doesn't mean other strains won't work. Stephanie Lay's autistic son, Bryce, now sixteen, is finally stable on a regimen of Marinol, a synthetic form of THC. I emailed Stephanie after reading about her advocacy online, then visited her in the wooded, lakeside Maine community where she lives, about ten minutes away from Bryce's group home. We sat in her living room while she showed me photos of some of the fourteen holes Bryce had put in the wall, mostly with his head. These violent behaviors had pre-cipitated seven psychiatric hospitalizations and three residential placements over the previous eight years. "The hardest part was wrestling with him after my double mastectomy, when I had three hundred stitches," Stephanie, a single mother, told me.[27]

Like virtually every other family I know, Stephanie tried count-less medications to control Bryce's behavior. "Nothing worked longer than three weeks," she said, until she got Bryce a prescrip-tion for medical marijuana and baked it into brownies. "He went five months without any behaviors. But then puberty happened. I'm no scientist—I had no idea how to adjust the dose to accom-modate his growth spurt." After his last hospitalization, doctors re-mained unconvinced it was safe for Bryce to return home. "It's very difficult for me that other people are helping me raise my child," Stephanie admitted. In fact, Bryce is with her almost as much as he's in the group home, coming back for three hours every after-noon and staying all weekend. Unfortunately, as much as Stepha-nie likes this placement, the staff is not permitted to administer the pot brownies. Marinol was the closest Stephanie could get.

"He's doing well," she told me, as the two of us waited with Bryce and the manager of his group home at a Mexican restaurant we had chosen for lunch. "He's been taking Marinol for almost two months, and he's only had two serious meltdowns."

The manager agreed. "We saw a significant increase in his abil-ity to self-regulate when the dose was increased from two to three times a day," she reported, but I could see for myself. As someone who would never have taken my son to a restaurant before he was medically stabilized without serious muscle (i.e., my husband, who, by the time Jonah was nine, was the only one who could still physi-cally manage his rages), I knew as soon as Stephanie accepted my in-vitation to lunch how well the Marinol must be working. And Bryce exhibited no disruptive behaviors the entire time we were together. He ate his order of french fries—Jonah's favorite food as well—and showed off his savant skill: being able to tell, given any date, what day of the week it would or did fall on. "What day will April 1, 2015 fall on?" I asked him in July 2014. "Wednesday," he said. I checked the calendar on my phone to confirm that he was right.

Stephanie has big plans for Bryce. "My goal is to have a house with a couple of acres, where he could have his own separate little cottage," she told me. She described a life filled with Bryce's favorite activities: surfing, swimming, horseback riding. "I think he's going to be fairly independent by the time he's in his twenties. He's learning how to cook—he makes macaroni and cheese, and uses the grill—and clean. He vacuums, does the laundry. I don't think he'll need full-time support."

But the cottage is for the future. Later that afternoon, after I left them, Stephanie told me she would be taking Bryce to the Goodwill store. He loves old VHS tapes so, as a reward, she often lets him pick one out for ninety-nine cents. I asked him what movie he wanted to pick out.

"*Peter Pan*," he said.

I found it incredibly poignant, for some reason: a wall of tapes in their worn cardboard sleeves; one boy in a tweed Sherlock Holmes cap perusing what I had to imagine was an extensive collection, fed by an entire community that had abandoned this antiquated technology. Such small pleasures, the ones our kids cherish most! I honestly hadn't realized you could buy VHS tapes anywhere, anymore.

AND WHAT ABOUT our experience with CBD oil?

The hemp derivative didn't help Jonah. His seizures kept increasing in frequency, until eventually we started him on an anticonvulsant. So far, the Onfi has completely stopped the episodes, with no apparent side effects.

But that doesn't mean I don't look at Jonah's complicated medical regimen and wonder what would have happened if marijuana had been available fifteen years ago, when his violent behaviors got him kicked out of the public school's autistic support kindergarten class and we started this long, tortuous road to stabilization. I have no doubt that I would have tried it first. I suppose I am a big believer in that old cliché: where there's smoke, there's fire. There are just too many reports of autistic kids whose symptoms have been reduced or even resolved after taking marijuana not to take those claims very seriously. Even many doctors concerned about possible side effects, like Kevin Gray, acknowledge the therapeutic possibilities: "I'm very supportive of research, no doubt about it," he told me. "We need to develop an evidence base and evaluate it accordingly."[28] Even Autism Speaks has taken notice: in November 2018, the organization hosted a two-day consensus conference on cannabis, featuring more than thirty stakeholders, including researchers, practitioners, and parents.[29] Although the classic joke about consensus conferences is that they are only held when consensus is lacking, the participants agreed with the wider call for more studies. It's too early to tell whether Autism Speaks has enough weight to provoke government action—to change marijuana's Schedule I classification, to license additional growers, to fund adequately powered research. All families in many states can do is wait.

6

All Possible Spaces

Amanda: One summer night, I took Jonah to one of the amusement piers in Ocean City, New Jersey. I was hoping he would skip past the Doubleshot, which was the only ride that agitated my otherwise very advanced vestibular system, but, no luck. Jonah spotted it. This ride, which I would have never chosen, since it essentially is like falling through a broken elevator, of course was what Jonah wanted to ride last. I knew he loved it though—the last shore trip I had gone with his whole family and his younger sister rode it with him. So I said OK, even though it seemed completely terrifying. We got in, we buckled our safety belts. As we prepared to be launched to the top of this tower, Jonah began to smile his big beautiful grin, giggle, and clap his hands in excited anticipation and I felt my fear melt away into joy because I knew I was going to experience one of those moments of sparkly happiness I loved to revel in with Jonah. When we got to the top, I remember seeing his face bathed in moonlight, his smile shining and then BAM! We quickly dropped to the bottom! His laughter became so loud, I experienced a brief second where the soundlessness of plummeting to the bottom of this ride was suddenly pierced with his very audible delight. I will never forget this particular moment as long as I live.[1]

Jonah's friendships are not like my other children's. With four neurotypical kids, I have a lot of experience watching these relationships develop—beginning when Erika was two and a half, when she came home from preschool and announced, "My best friend is Abby. She doesn't talk." Given that Erika never shut up, Andy and I observed to one another, this struck us as a particularly symbiotic arrangement.

Little kids make friends everywhere, easily. Marveling over Erika's (and later Hilary's, Aaron's, and Gretchen's) immediate and enthusiastic affection for new playmates from gymnastics, music class, school, or the playground, Andy would hypothesize to me how her mind must work: "You love candy? I love candy! Let's be best friends!" Developmental psychologists call this "Level 0 friendship"—the earliest in a five-stage progression from fleeting, fun encounters to stable, deeply emotional connections (acknowledging that these primitive forms of friendship can evolve—Erika and Abby, for example, are still best friends fifteen years later).[2]

Jonah has never had even level 0 friendships with other children. Not that we didn't try to facilitate them. When he was very small, we took him to toddler playgroups, Gymboree, and Sally's Music Circle. We asked our friends with children his age over to swim and bounce on the trampoline. Later, when he was in school, we invited his classmates to elaborate birthday celebrations featuring water slides and inflatable castles, and dutifully took Jonah to their parties.

How similar they were, those parties! Jonah is twenty years old now, and I suspect that, every weekend, parents of young autistic children throw them still: all with their gluten-free cupcakes, the carefully chosen gifts the children have no interest in opening, and the kids, completely ignoring one another, as if they have never met; each one chased by a parent as he or she scrambles through tunnels or bangs on arcade games at Chuck E. Cheese, because these venues always have so many exits, and all it takes is one distracted moment for a persistent eloper to disappear. At the time, though, it didn't feel like we were part of one big autism cliché. We were hopeful, and persistent, and we did it for many years, until one by one we all stopped.

Models like Robert Selman's five-level theory of friendship are based, of course, on neurotypical development—just like, more broadly, my assumptions about what friendship looks like were based on the interactions of my other children, as well as my memories of my own early relationships. For me—as, I imagine, for most people—friendship has always meant heads bent over board games or Barbies, seats saved in the cafeteria, inside jokes and sleepovers, late-night counseling sessions over phone or, today, text. Jonah's experience has been radically different. His most meaningful relationships have been with paid caregivers who have worked with him at home or school, which is why I wrote, in a piece for *Psychology Today*, that I thought he was "incapable of friendship."[3]

> *Kaitlin:* The Kermit Halloween costume is one of my favorite memories of working with Jonah. Nicole, Jannette and I had been working on a team together. As we spent time with Jonah, we saw many of his favorite clips from "Sesame Street" and "Elmo's World" played over and over. Halloween approached and we had the opportunity to bring our patients around the hospital trick-or-treating in different departments and offices. We knew that we wanted to have a Sesame Street character costume for Jonah, but Nicole quickly knew the clip for inspiration. Kermit the Gorf was a favorite because of the play on spelling, and probably Kermit's outrage and big reactions in the episode. Jonah had been drawing Kermit and writing out all the versions of the Kermit the Gorf/Forg/Grof in his very particular style of art. Nicole went out to purchase supplies for costumes including a green sweat suit with matching hat to put Kermit's eyes onto (for Jonah). She purchased t-shirts to make Kermit the FORG/

GORF/FROG shirts for the team using iron on letters. When we
came upstairs to the unit for trick-or-treating in our coordinating shirts, Jonah's face absolutely lit up and he looked shocked
too. I remember him checking out all of our shirts and the spelling on each shirt, and having a hard time standing in one place
to take a group photo because he was so excited.[4]

Developmental psychologists aren't the only ones who have
thought long and hard about friendship. Philosophers have wres-
tled with the definition and significance of this relationship since
Aristotle observed that "without friends no one would choose to
live." For him, friendship was one of the most sublime virtues—
one he believed inspired "noble actions," and could even "hold
states together."[5] Not surprisingly, given this account, he believed
that "perfect" friendship was only possible between men of the
most superior character.[6]

For Michel de Montaigne, writing at the end of the sixteenth
century, the key feature of friendship as he experienced it with
Étienne de la Boétie before the latter's untimely death was that it
was so all-consuming it precluded all other relationships. Montaigne describes "this friendship that possesses the whole soul, and
there rules and sways with an absolute sovereignty, [which] cannot possibly admit of a rival." Not even duties to wives, children,
or country take precedence: "A unique and particular friendship
dissolves all other obligations whatsoever."[7]

Obviously, Jonah is not capable of this kind of friendship. But I'm
not sure I am, either. I suspect Aristotle and Montaigne wouldn't
think so. They believed these highest forms of friendship were extraordinarily rare—Montaigne predicted a soul friendship like his
and La Boétie's might occur once every three hundred years.[8]

So what about the rest of us? Aristotle does acknowledge two
other types of friendship, based on utility and pleasure. For him,

these are inferior, or "incidental," relationships.[9] But contemporary philosophers have challenged this hierarchy, suggesting that such neat divisions may not be possible. Writes Alexander Nehamas, "It is not that our casual friendships are instrumental while our close ones are not: no friendship is purely instrumental but, also, no friendship is completely *un*instrumental."[10] For him, what is important is not the number or intensity of friendships, but their role in building the self—a project that is inherently relational and perpetually unfinished. His is a definition that resonates for me: "[Friends] influence what we do and how we understand it, how we understand ourselves, and what we are likely to become."[11]

> *Ben:* Jonah and I went on several overnight trips with school. The condo where we stayed had an outdoor pool where we spent a lot of time. Jonah loves when I throw him in the water. Over the years this activity has become increasingly difficult as Jonah is now taller than I am! Even if I can't throw him as far as I did when he was younger, I still do my best to keep this tradition alive. But even an entire day in the pool wasn't always enough to satisfy Jonah's desire for constant fun. One morning, he wanted to get an early start to the day and decided to wake me at 3:00 AM. I remember waking up and seeing Jonah in the doorway. He walked into my room, turned on the light, and said, "No light off. Ben gets up."[12]

It's nice to read that philosophers today no longer believe that friendship is only possible between archbishops and Supreme Court justices—but we've all figured that out by now. So why was I so quick to reject Jonah's relationships with paid caregivers as real friendships? I'm not the only one: disability rights advocates also draw a sharp line between friends and staff. In its position paper "Keeping the Promise: Self Advocates Defining the Meaning of Community Living," the Autistic Self Advocacy Network specifically defines "community" as a place where autistic people "integrate with people who don't have disabilities, and this does not mean staff."[13] The title of an article in the *Guardian* concisely sums it up: "People with Learning Disabilities Need Friends, Not Just Paid Carers."[14]

The most obvious obstacle is the money. A paid friend is like a jumbo shrimp, isn't it? A textbook example of an oxymoron. Caregivers aren't paid for their friendship, however—they're paid for their supervision, their instruction, their assistance. And I'm sure that many limit their involvement to exactly those things they're paid to do. But given the long hours spent together, and the often intimate circumstances, is it that surprising that deeper connections sometimes develop? The writer Donna Thomson notes this frequently happens with the caregivers employed to work with her son Nick, who has cerebral palsy: "Most of our paid caregivers over the years have remained close friends—some I would call lifelong best friends."[15] That's been our experience also—and not just with Jonah and his aides. All my kids are still very close to the nanny we had for seventeen years. The four youngest were attendants in her wedding, and even though she no longer works for us, she still hosts them for overnights, sends them flowers when they are sick or celebrating, and comes to their shows and ceremonies. Another old babysitter often takes my adventurous eaters to Philadelphia's Chinatown for spicy food, and Hilary's tutor gave her a framed montage of the goofy selfies they had taken during their sessions together for her bat mitzvah.

Besides, I hadn't written in my *Psychology Today* post, "Paid friendships are like jumbo shrimp." I had written, "Jonah is incapable of friendship." Obviously the real obstacle, for me, was the significant intellectual and developmental disability that precluded him from engaging in genuine social reciprocity. How many conversations had I had with my other kids about the importance of taking turns, of playing what their friends wanted to play even if they preferred a different game, of reaching out and being there? And also, less frequently but more heartbreaking: gently pointing out when their efforts and affections and invitations were not returned. "So-and-so is not a good friend," I would say. "You deserve so much better."

Jonah, it must be said, is all about Jonah. He never seems to think, "I wonder how Shaneen is feeling? What does Theresa want to do right now? How can I help?" His favorite adults—and they are always adults—don't mind. We know what he loves, and we reliably follow the script. We know how to make a "fun list," draw "Ernie half-a-hand," sing the "We all go home together" song (and then admit, under pressure from Jonah, that we "don't know what the 'We all go home together' song is"), and order lemonade with no ice. In return, we get . . . big smiles, sometimes sloppy kisses. It's more than enough, for us. But if Erika, Hilary, Aaron, or Gretchen came home from school and described a relationship that asymmetrical, I would caution, "That's not what real friendship is about."

But now I suspect that reciprocity may be for me what exclusivity and exceptionality were for Aristotle and Montaigne: a personal criterion that reveals more about me than it does about friendship as an institution. In their 2006 analysis of friendships in England, the sociologists Liz Spencer and Ray Pahl discovered that "the importance people attach to reciprocity varies enormously. . . . For [some people], reciprocity is less of a central concern. They accept that some friends are less able or less willing to contribute to the relationship, but find that the friendship has other qualities which are valued."[16] And it wasn't just reciprocity that differed. Spencer and Pahl had begun their research with the goal of defining friendship in the twenty-first century, but ultimately they gave up, concluding, "It is the very great diversity of ties, and the diversity of the circumstances or contexts that shape them, which provide the core finding of our study."[17] For them, friendships with co-workers, with neighbors, with siblings, with old schoolmates, even with professional help—they all counted.

> *Ashley:* One of my favorite times was slip-and-sliding with Jonah at Camp Joy. He wasn't on board at first but then exhausted us going up and down the hill to slide a million times—holding hands the whole time. But there are lots of other not distinct times that I loved hanging out with him. Most of them involved making up new silly songs or games to get him to keep jumping on the trampoline with me, or walk with me down the driveway, or reading a book while he fell asleep at bedtime.[18]

Jonah will attend his autistic support school until he's twenty-one. But, like many districts, ours begins planning for the transition to adult services at the age of fourteen. That's seven years to expose students to different jobs, with the hope of finding something that fits both interest and ability by the time they age out. If that seems like a long time, it's because work is of paramount importance to disability rights activists. Pennsylvania, where we live, is an "Employment First" state. According to the executive order Governor Tom Wolf signed in 2016, "The definition of Employment First is that competitive integrated employment is the first consideration and preferred outcome of publicly-funded education, training, employment and related services . . . for working-age Pennsylvanians with a disability" because work shapes "self-identity, self-worth and self-respect."[19]

Jonah has tried many jobs over the past six years. Even though I very much doubt he will ever be capable of competitive, minimum-wage work, he will still need activities to fill his days. So far, he has worked in restaurants, retirement communities, gyms, and offices. He's folded pizza boxes, watered plants, pulled weeds, wiped down equipment, rolled silverware, and stocked ice chests. He hasn't hated any of these gigs, but he hasn't loved any, either. I suspect he will do whatever task stands between him and his few preferred activities: watching his iPad, drawing, or best of all, dictating a "fun list" to a very enthusiastic, very patient scribe—which is why I've come to believe that, more than where he works or even where he lives, the single most important contributor to Jonah's quality of life will be the quality of his direct care staff.

Yet disability rights advocates are suspiciously silent on this issue. The National Council on Disability, for example, offers on its web page a long list of policy areas, including education, employment, and housing.[20] But I couldn't find any position statements or publications suggesting solutions to the direct care crisis currently facing not only the intellectually and developmentally disabled community, but all vulnerable populations. Staffing agencies across the country are reporting shortages as high as 30 percent, driven primarily by unlivable wages.[21] Earning an average of ten dollars an hour, almost half of direct care workers live below the poverty line.

Given this desperate need, agencies unsurprisingly require very few qualifications from applicants. Typically, a driver's license and a high school diploma are all that's required. And many states have no minimum training or supervision requirements. These factors in conjunction result in exactly the outcome you might expect. As mentioned earlier, as many as 90 percent of the intellectually and developmentally disabled experience abuse.[22] Just last month, I saw a familiar name in the headlines: two workers at a facility run by an agency that also operates a school Jonah attended when he was much younger were arrested for encouraging children to box and then posting the video on social media.

These incidents are met with predictable (and well-deserved) outrage. But the targets of that outrage often baffle me. Disability rights advocates frequently focus their blame on the size of some settings, or the degree of inclusion with the broader community, ignoring the most obvious and direct cause: behind every horrific act of abuse or neglect is a direct care worker who never should have been hired, not a building or a program. If there is one goal that the various disability communities should unite behind, one area of inarguable common ground, it's the need to build the strongest direct care workforce possible. Yet advocacy on this issue is spotty and localized. Last year, for example, Nicky's Law was proposed in Massachusetts to create a registry for abusive caregivers and prohibit agencies from hiring anyone on that list. But the bill was left languishing in the House when the legislative body disbanded for the summer.

> *Jessica:* Jonah still remembers, I believe, our very first trip to the water park almost five years ago. The whole way up, we made a list of what we were going to do: "white slide 130 more times, green slide 130 more times." Up one slide, down another. Over and over again until Jonah looked up and said "no slide." Just like that we were done, and he was ready to go. Finding a connection with someone like Jonah—knowing what to say and how to say it—is hard, and requires a deep knowledge of him. Honestly, you must study Sesame Street like a text book. But when you listen, and immerse yourself in his world, you're no longer just his teacher—you're his friend. And the thing about guys like Jonah—he's not being my friend to borrow my car or for me to loan him some money—he just likes me. We have a genuine connection that allows me to challenge him to be his best self, because he trusts me. Jonah isn't just one of my "students," he's

one of my friends. Even if we have to walk up and down the beach 130 times because there's nothing Jonah likes less than sitting still![23]

Jonah doesn't watch videos from beginning to end. He stops and starts, replaying fragments over and over. Sometimes the excerpts he chooses are so potent, so symbolic, that I can't help but wonder whether they reflect his innermost thoughts. Just this past weekend, Jonah kept listening to a song from the video *The Best of Ernie and Bert* about friendship. Before the music kicks in, Ernie and Bert are lying in their twin-size beds, when Ernie begins fretting about the toys he forgot to put away. Bert tells him not to worry about it, he can clean them up tomorrow, and Ernie says, "You know, Bert, you're a real friend. I'm messy and you don't like it messy, but because I'm your friend, you don't mind too much if I'm messy. That's what a friend is, Bert. Not minding too much because you like someone. . . . Not minding, that's what friends are for."[24]

Was Jonah thinking about friendship? "Jonah," I asked him, "who are your friends?" He didn't answer. I rephrased in different ways, trying to compensate for his difficulty with pronouns. "Bert is Ernie's friend," I said. "Who are Jonah's friends?"

When that didn't work either, I tried writing the question down, so Jonah could read it and write the answer. Jonah has significant auditory processing issues, so sometimes this increases the likelihood of getting a response. I wrote, "Ernie is Bert's friend. Who are Jonah's friends?" And I put a 1, 2, and 3 down the side of the page, hoping to engage Jonah's love of lists.

Next to the 1, he wrote, in his surprisingly careful print, "Ernie Is Bert's Friend."

Before he could continue, I took the marker out of his hand and had him read the top of the paper again: "'Ernie is Bert's friend.

Who are Jonah's friends?' Jonah, who are *Jonah's* friends? They can be people from home, or from school."

This is what Jonah wrote:

1. Bert's Friends Are Ernie
2. Jonah's Friends Are Who
3. Home

Maybe Jonah just likes that song for the tune, or the way Ernie dances around in a straw hat, then accompanies himself on the drums until Bert, in exasperation, goes to sleep in the kitchen. Maybe Jonah doesn't know what *friend* means. It wouldn't be that surprising, since, as Liz Spencer and Ray Pahl report, "it is clear that the word 'friend' encompasses a dizzying array of relationships"[25]—a particularly difficult concept for someone with minimal abstract language. But just because he can't define friendship doesn't mean he hasn't experienced it. Since I wrote that *Psychology Today* post, I've stopped comparing Jonah's friendships to mine, or his siblings', or classic cultural tropes like Tom and Huck, Sherlock and Watson, or Thelma and Louise. The fact that we use the same word to describe these bonds, as well as that of Montaigne and La Boétie, and even that of two-year-old Erika and Abby, reveals its immense breadth and generosity. As the philosopher Michel Foucault wrote about friendship, "We must think that what exists is far from filling all possible spaces."[26] Surely there is room, among all possible spaces, for Jonah and Nick, Jonah and Ky, Jonah and Jen—these friendships that Jonah considers as important and meaningful as my other kids count theirs.

Disability rights has always been about empowering the disabled to make their own choices—a critical mission that, I've repeatedly argued, fails to acknowledge the profound impairments of many individuals with severe intellectual and developmental disabilities.

Jonah can't make any decisions that require cost-benefit analyses, long-term projections, or immediate safety awareness. And what major decisions don't require these skills? He can't pick where he lives or works, or what type of medical or psychiatric treatment to pursue. He can't even decide to go to the mall for an Auntie Anne's pretzel by himself.

But Jonah can pick his friends. And he lets us know, all the time, about the special people in his life. He constantly presses his face to mine and says, "Waterpark with Ben and Jessica," or "Walk with Marina." His fun lists and pictures are peppered with people he hasn't seen in years: Melissa; Kaitlin, Nicole, and Jannette; Emily. Some names I don't even remember. Andy thinks Jackie and Jill may be teachers Jonah had when he was in preschool. Ultimately, what matters isn't whether these people were paid, whether these relationships were reciprocal, or whether anyone else would find them fulfilling. All that matters is that these bonds are important to Jonah.

Does this mean I no longer dream that, one day, Jonah will form a reciprocal friendship with a peer? No, I don't think I'll ever give that up. But that's now less about judging his relationships as lacking or inferior than it is part of a larger prayer that his world keeps expanding, that he has the opportunity to experience more and more of what this amazing world has to offer. I also know that, should this development ever occur, it will most likely be due to the very gentle, very persistent facilitation of an aide—the kind of committed, compassionate direct care worker that I hope, more than I do for anything else, will always be part of Jonah's life.

> *Nick:* The most fun thing I ever did with Jonah was take him to one of my favorite places, Wissahickon Creek Park. We walked along the path and Jonah let me know he was enjoying himself in the usual ways: jubilant outbursts, reciting some of his

favorite cartoon scenes, or looking at me eye to eye (literally). I knew he liked water so we walked down an old staircase built into the side of the bank of the creek down to a small waterfall. I was definitely nervous as I was normally good at anticipating Jonah's sometimes sudden moves, but this was a new place and we were standing near a waterfall and a creek. Even though it was fall, it was a warm day. What happened next? Jonah dropped down toward the ground in push-up position and gently put his lips to the cool, fall Wissahickon Creek water. He stood up and had the biggest smile on his face (and of course his t-shirt was soaked). We climbed back up to the gravel trail and headed out. It was a good day.[27]

7

Praesidalism

When words lose their customary meanings, Confucian thinkers urged, when they are applied recklessly to realities to which they weren't intended to apply, moral judgment melts away. Opportunists re-label bandits as kings and altruism as foolishness; sophists deviously twist meanings to make betrayal appear praiseworthy and recast righteousness as treachery. It is in this way that people lose their compass of superior and inferior, right and wrong, and chaos prevails. Indiscriminate language spawns wanton indiscrimination.

—*Shigehisa Kuriyama,* The Expressiveness of the Body

When you have a child with minimal language, it's easy, even necessary, to focus on the communicative function of language. "Hurt your eyes," Jonah says periodically, to me or to his teachers. Sometimes he says it while smiling and bouncing, but often he's crying, pressing his fists into his face. Since he reliably confuses his pronouns, I understand he is talking about himself, not me. "Does your head hurt?" I ask him. Somehow, we have come to think of these episodes as migraines. Jonah has punched through a window and seemed barely bothered by gashes in his hand held together by glue and tape ("Please, no stitches," I always begged the emergency room doctors, "he'll just pull them out"); he's suffered splinters the size of pencils while spinning shoeless on the Atlantic City Boardwalk and walked two miles back to our shore house without a limp. It's hard to imagine the level of pain that would make him cry. But migraines are just a guess. I give him ibuprofen, and sometimes it seems to help.

Language remains, in our house, a blunt instrument. All that matters is equipping Jonah with tools to express his preferences. Grammar, pronunciation—unimportant. We don't even care if the words are the right ones, so long as we're all in agreement. Often, we follow Jonah's lead: *white chips* are salt-and-vinegar potato chips; *nibbles* are the pink linings of rabbits' ears; *roll it chuck* is the dialogue bubble that pops up in children's programs— particularly, as far as Jonah is concerned, in a *Sesame Street* video called *Sing Yourself Sillier at the Movies.*

Perhaps that's why I was stunned when I first discovered how much vitriol was being exchanged online over whether to use the phrase "autistic person" or "person with autism." It's not that I'm unsympathetic to concerns with precision and connotation—as a writer, I've spent hours in front of my computer struggling to come up with the perfect word. But the difference between these two expressions just seemed so small. That hasn't stopped impassioned rhetoric from being deployed by both sides, however. *Person-first language* has been endorsed by the disability rights movement since the 1980s. "Most people do not like to be labeled," advises the Association of University Centers on Disabilities. "Therefore it is preferable to use people-first language [which] places the emphasis on the person instead of on the disability. . . . For example, instead of saying 'Down syndrome person,' it is preferable to say, 'person with Down syndrome.'"[1]

But many self-advocates take offense at such phrasing. Lydia Brown argues on her blog, *Autistic Hoya*, "When we say 'person with autism,' we say that it is unfortunate and an accident that a person is Autistic. . . . In fact, we are saying that autism is detrimental to value and worth as a person, which is why we separate the condition with the word 'with' or 'has.'" She, like many self-advocates, prefers *identity-first* language, such as "autistic person" or simply "autistic," because "we understand autism as an inherent part of an individual's identity—the same way one refers to 'Muslims,' 'African-Americans,' Lesbian/Gay/Bisexual/Transgender/Queer."[2]

These arguments frustrated me for many years. When you're spending every day trying to keep your kid from pulling out your hair or biting chunks out of your arm, the effort and indignation invested in a distinction that was (to me) so minor I could never remember which side was which seemed the petty and self-indulgent purview of people with way too much time on their hands. I planted myself firmly with autism parent and blogger Stuart Duncan, in his "I don't care group": "I don't take sides. It's ridiculous. Seriously, is this how we want to spend our time? Is terminology really a reason to get mad at each other? Can something this childish really begin to divide a community?"[3]

But in the eight years since he wrote that post, it's become clear that, to answer Duncan's questions: yes, seriously, language wrangling is how many people want to spend their time; it is a reason that people get mad at each other; and it does continue to divide the autism community. Not just over the *autistic* vs. *person with autism* question. I think my hang-up with that particular controversy kept me from seeing how many loaded words there are in this field—phrases that have tremendous impact on public and private perceptions of autism, the specific supports and services offered to this population, and our overall societal approach to dependency and care. I can't think of another reason why it took me so long to figure it out. The notion that language is important and consequential is so ubiquitous that I recently stumbled upon it—not in a book about autism, or disability in general, but about the nineteenth-century British botanist Joseph Hooker: "Language is not a neutral medium for conveying facts but a complex method of persuasion."[4] As far as I'm concerned, if you run into the same idea in both contemporary disability blogs and texts assigned for your Colonial Botany seminar, you can pretty much accept it as a universal truth.

Autism/Asperger's

When we first met with a developmental pediatrician sixteen years ago, I wasn't sure what diagnosis Jonah would get. It was obvious he was on the spectrum by that point, but where? Since he wasn't talking, I knew he didn't have Asperger's syndrome—that label was for kids with no intellectual disability or speech delays. I also knew he didn't have Rett syndrome (which only affects girls) or childhood disintegrative disorder (which describes kids who experience a late and significant regression in skills). But would the doctor tell us Jonah had autism, or pervasive developmental disability, not otherwise specified (PDD/NOS)? I knew that PDD/NOS, otherwise known as "autism lite," was a muddy category that could reflect a moderate range of functioning, or simply a doctor's desire to spare anxious parents. Still, I rooted for it—although he didn't get it. Jonah was only two years old, but I had already figured out that in the community of parents, therapists, and doctors, the distinctions between Asperger's, autism, and PDD/NOS were important and useful.

Today, all children on the spectrum get the same diagnosis: autism spectrum disorder. In 2013, the American Psychiatric Association revised its *Diagnostic and Statistical Manual of Mental*

Disorders (*DSM-5*), officially eliminating familiar diagnoses, including Asperger's and PDD/NOS. Autism now includes a staggering range of disability—represented by Dr. Shaun Murphy from *The Good Doctor* on one end, to anonymous cognitively impaired, nonverbal and self-injurious individuals on the other, who have never been, and will never be, featured in any television show.

The logic behind the changes seemed sound. "There wasn't any evidence after 17 years that [the *DSM-IV* diagnoses] reflected reality," says Bryan King, director of Seattle Children's Autism Center, who served on the association's task force charged with revamping the diagnosis. "There was no consistency in the way Asperger's or PDD-NOS was applied."[5] In fact, a 2011 study by Catherine Lord (another member of the task force) and more than thirty-five colleagues reported, "In these 12 university-based sites, with research clinicians selected for their expertise in ASD and trained in using standardized instruments, there was great variation in how best-estimate clinical diagnoses within the autism spectrum (i.e., autistic disorder, PDD-NOS, Asperger's disorder) were assigned to individual children."[6] In other words, the diagnoses children received depended largely on where they were diagnosed.

While these diagnoses may be, on the margins, somewhat arbitrary, they are absolutely not meaningless to the autism community. When the American Psychiatric Association proposed the new classification system, it was met with much protest; more than 8,000 people signed an online petition circulated by the Global and Regional Asperger's Syndrome Partnership; another petition sponsored by Asperger's Association of New England received 5,400 signatures. So-called Aspies argue that the word "autism" carries a greater stigma, which may keep high-functioning individuals and their families from pursuing a diagnosis and the support that comes with it. As high-school senior Hannah Fjeldsted, who has Asperger's, articulated clearly (if a bit insensitively) in a guest blog at Autism Speaks, "The label of Asperger's at least gives observers the impression of intelligence and ability. But when most people think of 'autism,' they think of someone who should be institutionalized."[7] Tom Hibben, author of the *Adventures in Asperger's* blog, wonders whether his son will embrace the new diagnosis. "Now it's almost cool to have Asperger's," he points out. "*The Big-Bang Theory* and *Parenthood* feature characters who have it."[8]

Parents of severely autistic kids were also not thrilled to welcome much more mildly afflicted individuals, with their very different support needs, into a diagnosis that has historically—as Hannah Fjeldsted pointed out—represented significant disability. One mother commented online that "it does a disservice to the people with severe or classic autism to lump them with aspergers and high functioning persons. It gives the public a distorted perception of what autism is. It is crippling to my son and many like him."[9] Judith Ursitti, director of state and government affairs for Autism Speaks and mother of a child on the spectrum, has similar concerns: "If we have this national perspective that autism is a blessing, that it's not a crisis, the ones who will lose out are the expensive ones, the severe ones. Legislators focus on the cheapest option, and celebration is cheaper than treatment."[10]

It's not just parents—many professionals also believe in the old diagnostic distinctions. Simon Baron-Cohen, director of the Autism Research Center at the University of Cambridge, hypothesized in a 2009 *New York Times* editorial that Asperger's may be a biologically distinct syndrome; his team identified fourteen genes that might be associated with the condition.[11] A 2012 study of more than 540 Australian health and education professionals found that 93 percent thought there was a real difference between autism and

Asperger's. Just over half the respondents were opposed to the consolidation of the diagnoses, while less than a quarter supported it.[12] University of Michigan psychiatrist Luke Tsai analyzed almost 130 studies comparing autism and Asperger's and found that almost 100 of them "concluded that there were statistically significant or near significant levels of quantitative and/or qualitative differences between [Asperger's and autism]" as well as "more than ninety clinical variables that have been investigated and have demonstrated that they can be used to show the significant differences."[13] His prediction? As he titled his article, "Asperger's Disorder Will Be Back."

If it does return, it will reflect the growing consensus that there is no one disease entity called autism. The Canadian geneticist Stephen Scherer has referred to "the many 'autisms' that make up the autism spectrum."[14] Caltech neuroscientist Ralph Adolphs described his research as an "initial step in trying to discover what kinds of different autisms there actually are."[15] And a report from the 2013 International Meeting for Autism Research highlighted "the idea of autism vs. 'autisms'" as a pervasive theme of the conference.[16]

It seems so simple and obvious—carve the spectrum back up, as writer and autism parent Marie Myung-Ok Lee proposed in *Salon* in 2014: "Separat[e] the high-functioning end of the spectrum—perhaps call it something else—so that we can focus on the urgent and looming issue at hand."[17] Besides Asperger's, maybe we could also introduce a new diagnosis for the most impaired—those with autism, intellectual disability, and minimal or no language. My vote is Kanner syndrome, named for Leo Kanner, who, along with Hans Asperger, is credited with separately discovering autism and who documented cases of children more profoundly affected than Asperger's patients.

I'm actually surprised we have to defend this type of classification, which is standard in other disorders that—like autism—fall along a broad continuum. Many people have varying degrees of visual impairment, but only those at the tail end of the spectrum are blind. Those individuals who meet clinical definitions of deafness or obesity certainly share commonalities with those who are hard of hearing or overweight, but the severity of these cases necessitates greater support and intervention, and everyone easily appreciates those differences.

Not only would this change clarify matters for the general public, but I really believe it would bring peace to the enormous and deeply divided autism community. As noted, autistic self-advocates and parents of severely autistic children are constantly at war over whether or not autism should be cured and what educational, vocational and residential services should be provided with our always limited local and federal budgets. Separating out these diagnoses would let those affected by each pursue the most appropriate agenda for that population, which seems like a win for everybody.

High Functioning/Low Functioning

At first glance, the high-functioning/low-functioning binary seems like just another version of the autism/Asperger's debate. And while it's true that these categories map to some extent— Asperger's is typically cast as the high-functioning end of the spectrum—these labels deploy different politics. No one denies the need for diagnostic terms. Research and advocacy efforts focus on how many are appropriate, and how to quantify them, but I've yet to hear anyone call for the dismantling of the entire apparatus. Yet I can think of few things more certain to incite a digital riot than the descriptors *high functioning* and *low functioning*.

Autistic self-advocates in particular are quick to reject the division of the spectrum along this axis. Lydia Brown believes all autistics "suffer from these arbitrary, hurtful labels" which "only describe ideas that don't exist in reality" and "reek of ableism . . . paternalism [and] laziness." Despite the fact that her college education and her advocacy work lead many to observe as much, Brown emphatically states, "I don't feel 'high-functioning.'"[18] Cynthia Kim puts it most succinctly on her blog, *Musings of an Aspie*, opining that she herself is "'high functioning' one moment and 'low functioning' the next."[19]

While Brown is right that *high functioning* and *low functioning* "don't even describe precise or definite ideas"—if she's referring to the lack of objective criteria, such as IQ score, or ratings on various assessments of language or adaptive living skills—I have never heard anyone described as low functioning who didn't have a significant intellectual disability. Students at prestigious universities (like Brown) and wives, mothers, and successful entrepreneurs (like Kim) are simply not low functioning, even if they procrastinate on their homework or need to be reminded to brush their hair—examples Brown and Kim give of their "nonlinear" functioning. These persistent efforts to recast functioning as a "fluid" dimension (Kim's descriptor) only end up co-opting those who, like Jonah, are absolutely crippled by autism, into an advocacy effort that reflects the goals of a much more privileged population.

Parents of severely autistic kids are quick to remind self-advocates of this privilege; as Jennifer Franklin Nash said in an article in *New York* magazine, "I'd like nothing more than for [my daughter] to develop the kind of consciousness that would allow her to join the neurodiversity movement."[20] Feda Almaliti wryly adds, in a blog for the Autism Society of San Francisco, "Heck, if [my son] attended a conference about autism discrimination he'd be kicked out in two minutes."[21]

So many parents have raised this point, this locus of difference between their voiceless children and the autistic self-advocates, that Julia Bascom, deputy executive director for the Autistic Self Advocacy Network, felt compelled to respond. But rather than acknowledge that cognitive disparity and all its implications on educational and vocational achievement, communication, independence, and overall quality of life, her 2011 blog post "Dear 'Autism Parents'" simply denies it. To parents who tell her, "If my child could write a blog post like this, I would consider him cured," Bascom has this to say:

> Fascinating. Have you taught him how? Have you given him the time, tools, technology, and accommodations he would need to do so? Have you exposed him to the ideas this blog post runs on, or has he been sheltered and infantilized? Has he been given an accessible, for him as well as his audience, means of communication? . . . Have multiple literacies been facilitated? Remember, *everyone reads, everyone writes, everyone has something to say* is the current forward-thinking in special education, especially for children with complex access needs. But you're an advocate for your child, of course you must know that. Silly me, I apologize.[22]

What is so notable about this excerpt—besides its peerless contempt—is that Bascom really seems to believe that the only reason profoundly autistic individuals aren't articulating insightful ideas is that their parents have failed them. She just doesn't accept that there are those whose significant intellectual disability precludes the level of abstract thinking, logical reasoning, and creative processing necessary to make any kind of philosophical argument, never mind write a blog post. Consider Jonah:

"Have you taught him how?" We didn't have to teach Jonah to write; he taught himself before he learned how to talk.

"Have you given him the time, tools, technology, and accommodations he would need to do so?" Of course. Not only does he have stacks of paper and markers in his room, but he uses a computer, an iPad, and an iTouch. It's amazing how fast he can type on that little screen, even though his fingers are perpetually swollen after years of pounding—on himself, on us, on hard surfaces like floors, walls, windows.

"Have you exposed him to the ideas this blog post runs on?" No. Jonah's capacity for abstract thought is very limited. That is not "infantilizing" him; it is just the way he is, like so many of those at the severe end of the spectrum. The types of texts we read with him in our constant quest to expand his comprehension are very simple stories, not political treatises. "Jonah, listen," I might say. "The girl went to her grandmother's farm to pick apples. What did the girl pick at her grandmother's farm? Jonah?" To which he might answer, "farm" or "girl," or maybe, after much prompting, "apples," which would catapult me out of my chair in excitement.

"Remember, everyone reads, everyone writes, everyone has something to say." It is simply untrue that everyone reads and writes. I know families whose autistic children struggle to identify simple shapes and colors. Fortunately, Jonah can read and write. He almost exclusively writes lists, that only resemble lists as we understand them because of their numbered entries, like "1. N N" and "30. Mommy draws big bird and Yeah." Bascom is right in that Jonah has plenty to say: "No school," "*Big* orange juice," "Mommy and Daddy leave and Jonah stays at Costco" (so he can ransack the bakery department). And after waiting for more than a decade for him to express more abstract thoughts and ideas, I've finally come to accept that what he writes and says pretty accurately reflects what he's thinking.

Despite attacks like Bascom's, parents persist in demanding that the autism community pay attention to their profoundly disabled children. As I was working on this essay, Facebook alerted me to a "fiery exchange" that erupted at the October 24, 2017, meeting of the Interagency Autism Coordinating Committee (IACC), which advises the National Institute of Health how to spend their autism research dollars. As Sara Luterman reported for the online NOS Magazine—which describes itself as "a news and commentary source for thought and analysis about neurodiversity culture and representation"—Jill Escher, the president of the Autism Society of San Francisco and the parent of two severely autistic children, submitted a public comment "complain[ing] that neurodiversity has ruined the validity of autism as a diagnosis because it includes 'high functioning' people like the autistic representatives on IACC and 'low functioning' people like her own children. This sparked a tense conversation among members of IACC."[23]

And still, autistic self-advocates keep shifting the conversation. Instead of high or low functioning, they prefer to consider "need"—as in this retort to Escher from Samantha Crane, the director of public policy at the Autistic Self Advocacy Network (and a graduate of Harvard Law School): "We strongly believe that people with significant needs need to be empowered to also speak for themselves. . . . If we had people on the IACC who have significant communication needs and people on the IACC who have significant independent living support needs, the IACC might look different."[24]

Crane completely ignores Escher's main point: her children *cannot* speak for themselves. This isn't a question of empowerment, but one of significant cognitive impairment. That's the problem with replacing "functioning" with "need" as a descriptor: they're not synonymous. Christopher Reeve had very high support needs; so did Stephen Hawking. Yet these in no way affected their intellect or insight. In fact, the power and eloquence of Reeve and Hawking and other physically disabled advocates like John Hockenberry and Joni Eareckson Tada helped shape public acceptance, even expectation, of the disabled agency that Crane so passionately promotes—a development long overdue that should be unquestionably celebrated. All Escher—and Nash and Almaliti and I—are asking is that our low-functioning children not be syntactically erased from the conversation in the name of advancing that celebration.

Paternalism

Some words are not, exclusively on the basis of their dictionary definitions, particularly controversial, yet the baggage they have accumulated makes them irredeemable. *Asylum* is one such word; in 2015, the University of Pennsylvania ethics professors Dominic Sisti, Andrea Segal, and Ezekiel Emanuel ignited a firestorm when they argued, in an editorial in the *Journal of the American Medical Association*, that we need to "bring back the asylum." I interviewed Sisti for an article I wrote about residential options for autistic adults[25] because, although his paper focused on the care of patients with chronic psychiatric disorders, his description of individuals "who cannot live alone, cannot care for themselves, or are a danger to themselves and others" reminded me of Jonah.[26]

Sisti regretted using the word *asylum*: "We were trying to rehabilitate the term, bring it back to its original meaning, which is a place of sanctuary and healing," Sisti told me. But *asylum* has become too wedded to ghastly images of custodial institutions (another word that is beyond redemption, at least in this context; you can still describe Harvard as an institution, but you can't argue that your severely autistic child has intense support needs that would be best served in an institution). In the end, Sisti said, it was too distracting: "Everyone focused on that instead of the ethical imperative, which is clear: we need settings that match up with each individual's needs."[27]

Paternalism is, in some ways, harder to defend than *asylum*—the offensive ideas are built right into the word. The Latin root *pater* makes it explicitly sexist in its conceptual claim that father knows best, but not mother—an odd bias, when you remember that the vast bulk of caregiving work has historically been and continues to be done by women. Additionally, modeling care on the parent-child relationship is obviously infantilizing to the recipient. No wonder that one of the most withering dismissals made by disability rights activists about a particular policy or program is that it is paternalistic; Harlan Hahn calls paternalism "perhaps the most serious and intractable hindrance to the advancement of the rights of people with disabilities" and "an even more formidable obstacle in the struggle for equality than direct conflict or even hostility."

It's not just the semantically objectionable terminology that bothers Hahn. Inherent in his argument that paternalism "appears not only to justify the powerful position of nondisabled persons but also to conceal the comparatively powerless status of the disabled minority" is his belief that paternalism is purely political. Nowhere does he acknowledge the possibility that certain very vulnerable and cognitively incapacitated populations require lifelong protection and care. Even when he writes about the intellectually disabled, Hahn relies on sweeping generalizations about individuals who can "shap[e] their own destiny or challeng[e] the decisions made on their behalf by spokespersons from the dominant segment of society."[28]

Sound familiar? That inspiring, if sadly incomplete, rhetoric could have been written by Julia Bascom or Lydia Brown. So many issues plaguing severely cognitively impaired individuals and their families originate in this blinkered approach to disability rights, this refusal to see Jonah and all his complex, human, yet persistently dependent peers. This deliberate blindness is not new. Thirty years ago, Philip Ferguson called out the "pattern of de facto exclusion" of the severely intellectually disabled by the disability rights movement. This was "not simply an oversight or an understandable delay," he wrote, "[but] a logical concomitant of the conceptual base"—which locates deficit in our unaccommodating society (the social model of disability), not in individual bodies (the medical model of disability). Ferguson concludes, "If the disability rights movement is ever to achieve an inclusive vision of the future for all people with disabilities, then it must first open its eyes to the mistakes and triumphs of the past."[29]

Three decades later, the disability rights movement is no closer to "an inclusive vision of the future" that respects the diverse and intensive needs of the profoundly cognitively impaired. At the United Nations World Autism Awareness Day celebration in March 2017, the then chair of the Committee on the Rights of Persons with Disabilities, Theresia Degener, argued that guardianship law "must be repealed," comparing it to "slavery" and "genital mutilation."[30] Her statement—baffling and offensive to parents whose adult children, like Jonah, can't cross the street unsupervised—is completely consistent with the United Nations Convention on the Rights of Persons with Disabilities. As the Columbia professor Paul Appelbaum has noted, this committee has already decreed that "legal capacity is a universal attribute inherent in all persons by virtue of their humanity" and that "the existence of an impairment . . . must never be grounds for denying legal capacity."

Consider this truly stunning statement: Jonah has legal capacity—because the United Nations says so. End of story. His lack of abstract language, his inability to understand concepts such as money, property, voting—all that is dismissed with the magic of a mandate that might seem well-intentioned, but in actuality, as Appelbaum points out, "urge[s] abandonment of those persons most in need of protection. . . . People with severe disabilities also have rights to protection from the consequences of their conditions."[31]

Scholars from different disciplines—including philosophy, women's studies, bioethics, and sociology—have increasingly articulated this right to protection as an ethic of care that would supplement or even replace traditional liberalism's emphasis on autonomy. The focus shifts from the individual to the relation; as the psychologist Carol Gilligan defined it in a 2011 interview, "the ethics of care starts from the premise that as humans we are inherently relational, responsive beings and the human condition is one of connectedness or interdependence."[32] Agrees Eva Feder Kittay, "We have to use our multiple voices to expose [this] fiction [of autonomy] and rebuild a world spacious enough to accommodate us all with our aspirations of a just and caring existence."[33]

We may all need care, but most of us will be able to articulate our preferences, make important decisions, and report abuse. Kittay, from her unique position as both a philosopher and a parent of an adult child with significant cognitive impairments, has done perhaps more than any other scholar to apply the ethics of care to the severely intellectually disabled, whose ability to participate is qualified or even nonexistent. She champions the need for caregivers "genuinely, perhaps uniquely, concerned with the well-being of the dependent."[34] While parents most obviously fit this description, Kittay extends this qualification to the paid attendants who inevitably end up supporting intellectually disabled children and adults in their schools, day programs, and residential settings. In an industry marked by meager wages, minimal qualifications, and high turnover, this is a radical claim—one that demands an overhaul of policies regulating care. For Kittay, that includes ensuring that caregivers earn a living wage and are provided with health-care, paid vacation days, and possibly even housing.

As we lobby for these supports, I think it would be useful to attach a name to this ethic of care. Kittay suggests *doulia* to define a society-wide system of support for caregivers, both familial and paid: "Just as we have required care to survive and thrive, so we need to provide conditions that allow others—including those who do the work of caring—to receive the care they need to survive and thrive."[35] She derives the term from *doula*, which refers to a person who attends a woman in labor, then cares for her while she tends to her new baby.

I love Eva Feder Kittay, but I suspect that *doulia* will never catch on. Like *paternalism*, it evokes parent-child relationships (only connoting mothers instead of fathers), infantilizing the dependent person. Additionally, its very gendered connotation with women's work could easily alienate half the population. The point is that we *all* move in and out of dependent states and that we all need to value the work of caring for our most vulnerable citizens.

Instead, I suggest *praesidalism*, from the Latin *praesideo*, which means "to keep watch or stand guard over." There are other Latin synonyms we could borrow—*custodio, tuto, curato, protectio*—but these roots are pervasive in English, automatically evoking loaded words like *cure* and *custody*. Or we could consider Greek: *prostasia, egnoia, skotoura*. I don't really care what we call it—except I will admit a preference for something that sounds important and consequential. Something deserved, not given begrudgingly. Something that we as a country take seriously, as one of our most basic responsibilities, like education or national security. Imagine it as part of the Department of Health and Human Services: *assistant secretary for praesidalism*. You can tell just from the weight of it that it would be a privilege to serve.

So does any of this mean that I've adopted *autistics* over *people with autism*? It certainly means I think about the choices I'm making whenever I use those words—which, as you might imagine, is frequently. I happen to agree with self-advocates like Lydia Brown that autism is "an inherent part" of Jonah's identity—although I'm skeptical that the general public infers much difference in meaning between such similar-sounding and equally respectful terms as *autistic* and *person with autism*. Ultimately, I've come to believe that people should decide for themselves what they would like to be called, and since Jonah has no preference, I try to respect those who do—even as I resist efforts by some autistics to shift public perception through other strategic language choices that sanitize severe autism.

The French philosopher Sandra Laugier argues that language is inseparable from care: "Our ethical preoccupations are embedded in our language and our life, in clusters of words that extend beyond our ethical vocabulary itself and sustain complex connections with a variety of institutions and practices." She summarizes, "Language affects us, allows us to affect others, and constantly transforms our meanings."[36] So when a friend of mine, a fellow parent of a profoundly autistic child, describes our kids as "high need," I stop her. I ask her why she chose that particular phrase, which I'd never heard her use before. I ask her if she thinks it's precise and accurate, what other descriptors she could have chosen. I ask her to consider who sets the terms of the debates that currently divide the autism community, and more generally, our wider polity. I stop shy of inviting her down that rabbit hole where *Kanner Syndrome* and *praesidalism*, *low-functioning* and *institution* and *Asperger's* and *asylum* collect with all our other imperfect words past, present, and future. It's a mind trip, honestly. You never know what you will find, once you're down there.

8

The Child Who Does Not Know How to Ask

The Torah describes four children who ask questions about the Exodus. Tradition teaches that these verses refer to four different types of children.

The wise child asks, "What are the laws that God has commanded us?" The parent should answer by instructing the child in the laws of Passover, starting from the beginning and ending with the laws of the Afikomen.

The wicked child asks, "What does this Passover service mean to you?" The parent should answer, "It is because of what God did for me when I came out of Egypt. Specifically 'me' and not 'you.' If you had been there (with your attitude), you wouldn't have been redeemed."

The simple child asks, "What is this Seder service?"

The parent should answer, "With a mighty hand God brought us out of Egypt. Therefore, we commemorate that event tonight through this Seder."

And then there is the child who does not know how to ask.

—*Jewish Federations of North America,*
The Passover Haggadah

We were not a very observant family, growing up. We had a seder every year, but the joke was that each new reader would skip forward a few paragraphs in the Haggadah, the book that relates the story of the Exodus, to get to the meal faster—which in itself was not actually kosher for Passover, since my mother didn't observe the dietary restrictions of the holiday or see why they should preclude her from serving her famous noodle pudding.

But I remember the parable of the four sons (as it was called before modern theologians adopted the more politically correct "children"). I remember identifying with the wise son—not because of his desire to be instructed in the laws of Judaism, which held little interest for me, but because, as an awkward and lonely child, I liked to see the smart kid come in first. And I remember assuming that "the child who does not know how to ask" must be a baby or young toddler. Didn't the "simple" child already represent those with learning differences or intellectual disabilities? Was there anything worse?

I didn't know then that I would have a severely autistic son who would "not know how to ask"—not because he couldn't talk, because he can to some degree, but because he doesn't understand abstract concepts like God and faith, life and death, past and future. I didn't know that while my four other kids attended Hebrew school, preparing for the bar and bat mitzvah services that would celebrate their acceptance, at age thirteen, as Jewish adults, Jonah would stay home, working with the countless therapists we engaged to somehow stop him from pounding himself in the face, attacking us, punching out windows, and taking off alone down our busy road in the amount of time it took to answer the phone or pour a glass of milk. I didn't know that while our extended family gathered at our house for the seder every spring, we would let

Jonah watch *Sesame Street* videos in his room, because the frustration of sitting at the table and waiting for food while we read and sang through the adapted Haggadah we stole from the kids' Jewish preschool inevitably led to uncontrollable rages.

That's not what you're supposed to do with "the child who does not know how to ask," of course. The parable advises that "the parent should begin a discussion with that child based on the verse: 'And you shall tell your child on that day, "We commemorate Passover tonight because of what God did for us when we went out of Egypt.'"[1] But when your child doesn't understand "Passover" or "God" or "Egypt," when he has no comprehension of history or symbolism or tradition, you might wonder, as I did for many years, What's the point?

NOTHING IS MORE incompatible with God than severe intellectual disability. God is the ultimate abstraction, definable only by other abstractions: incorporeal, eternal, omniscient. Impossible to grasp by a mind so literal that when I once told Jonah, "Write your name on this birthday card for Grandma Judi," he very carefully printed, "YOUR NAME."

But even more difficult is the challenge severe intellectual and developmental disability poses for the Judeo-Christian belief in a just and merciful God. Why would he create humans who could never know him? How is that degree of cognitive impairment "in his image," or consistent with his demands for complex and particular ritual observance (in the Old Testament) and self-sacrifice (in the New Testament)?

Perhaps that's why there's no one like Jonah in the Bible. I started my search in the Haggadah, even though it's not actually part of the Bible, because I remembered the reference to "the child who does not know how to ask." After that turned out to be a dead end—scholars generally agree this child is neither young nor dull, but merely uninterested—I read both the Old and New Testaments. I was looking for a point of entry, an embrace—or if not an embrace, at least an acknowledgment—across the centuries of Jonah and his significant disabilities. But I found nothing.

Disability is seldom even addressed in the Old Testament. Moses allegedly suffered from a speech impediment, but it obviously didn't slow him down too much. There's a token directive not to "insult the deaf, or place a stumbling block before the blind" (Lev. 19:19)[2], but that is belied by the treatment of the few disabled people mentioned in the text. God in fact prohibits any of Aaron's descendants with a "defect" from entering the priesthood, which is basically the family business. And any man with one particular impairment (involving his privates, if you must know) is barred from the congregation altogether. "The lame and the blind" are explicitly called out as "hateful to David," who directs his soldiers to "strike [them] down" (2 Sam. 5:8). Even the animals offered for sacrifice must be, as it is hammered over and over again, "without blemish" (Exo 29:1).

The New Testament, by contrast, is full of disabled people. In every other verse, it seems, Jesus is healing someone else: "The blind are recovering their sight, cripples are walking again, lepers being healed, the deaf hearing, dead men are being brought to life again" (Luke 7)[3]. But these disabilities are almost exclusively physical or sensory, not intellectual. My hope briefly flared after encountering one figure whose dangerous behaviors evoked challenges frequently associated with profound intellectual and developmental disability. He "had worn no clothes for a long time and did not live inside a house"; for his own safety, he was "bound with chains and fetters and closely watched," but he would "snap his bonds and go off into the desert" (Luke 8). However, this man is completely articulate, and able to ask quite clearly—even in the midst of possession by evil spirits, the diagnosis made by his contemporaries—"What have you got to do with me, you Jesus, Son of the Most High God? Please, please, don't torment me." Given his ability to pose such a question, it seems likely this man's diagnosis today would be psychosis, not intellectual disability.

But maybe I shouldn't be too disappointed in the Bible's apparent lack of inclusion. It's not obvious there were many people like Jonah around during ancient times. In some cities, like Sparta, infants with any obvious disability were killed at birth. But even in somewhat more tolerant societies, the disability scholar Ellis Craig notes, "People with severe intellectual impairments, often with concomitant medical issues, probably did not live long, given the absence of medical treatment."[4] Biblical writers can hardly be faulted for excluding members of a population they rarely, if ever, encountered.

This silence hasn't stopped modern authors from interpreting cognitive impairments through a Biblical lens. Disabilities in general are blamed on "the fall of humankind into sin" and considered "a *normal* part of life in an *abnormal* world."[5] But despite this punitive origin, many writers argue that disability confers tremendous advantages. The theologian Larry Waters argues,

> Suffering produces knowledge and teaches God's will. Suffering teaches the sufferer to look to future glory and to learn obedience and self-control. Suffering teaches patience and perseverance, and encourages a life of faith. Suffering helps the sufferer to understand God's gracious purpose, to share in Christ's suffering and represent him to others, and to pray and give thanks in time of trouble. Suffering can glorify God, deepen one spiritually, and teach humility and contentment. The ultimate objective . . . is to lead the sufferer to a deeper understanding of a true relationship with Yahweh, the definitive teacher.[6]

Or, as disability advocate Joni Eareckson Tada sums it up, in an imagined conversation directly with God, "I do not think I would ever have known the glory of your grace were it not for the weakness of that wheelchair."[7]

Sounds like a pretty good deal, right? A (relatively) brief period of suffering in exchange for eternal life. But what if the sufferer's cognitive impairments are so profound they preclude any of the prayer and thanksgiving and other hard work required to earn those heavenly rewards? Unfortunately, none of the theologians I read believed that suffering alone was sufficient. The believer's response to suffering—the Job-like faith that persists even through the most grueling ordeals—is of paramount importance.

Perhaps that's why books about religion and intellectual disability tend to focus instead on the benefits to caregivers—a theme of virtually every parent memoir I read. "The veil has been lifted from my eyes, and I now see beauty where I used to see emptiness," writes Kelly Langston about life with her autistic son, Alec. "There is compassion in me where there once was selfishness. There is laughter and fun where there used to be a constant mental rundown of tasks yet to be completed. There is even personal acceptance instead of feelings of inadequacy. I would not trade these gifts for the world."[8] Kathy Medina, another mother of an autistic son, reminds her readers, "God is going to do what it takes for us to build our character."[9]

I don't disagree. There's no doubt that raising Jonah has brought a greater sense of purpose to my life, has stripped it of (most) petty concerns, and has crystallized all my murky allegiances. Steeling myself against Jonah's violent attacks; persisting in teaching him language; scrambling to stay one step ahead of his constant plotting to walk five miles to the mall, empty an entire jar of jelly beans onto the counter, or throw his iPad out the window; fighting to place him in the best schools—and, when the time came, the most respected inpatient unit in the country—has so greatly increased my strength, my wisdom, and (paradoxically, perhaps) my serenity that I feel alienated in many ways from my younger self.

It's not just me. Andy is more flexible and patient; our four other children are more empathetic and inclusive. There's no doubt that Jonah has made us all better people. But to suggest this somehow compensates for his purposeless suffering, missed experiences, and complete dependence implies a disturbingly instrumental view of human life that culminates in the 1988 narrative *The Power of the Powerless: A Brother's Legacy of Love*, Christopher De Vinck's account of his brother Oliver, who spent his entire thirty-two years lying silently in his bed, "blind, mute. His legs were twisted. He didn't have the strength to lift his head or the intelligence to learn anything. Oliver was born with severe brain damage that left his body in a permanent state of helplessness." Yet, De Vinck states, this "tragedy was turned into a joy. . . . He evoked the best love that was in us. He helped us to grow in the virtues of devotion, wisdom, perseverance, kindness, patience and fidelity."[10]

I don't blame De Vinck and his family for seeing the best in this utterly heartbreaking situation: while she was pregnant with Oliver, De Vinck's mother was found unconscious from a gas leak, which presumably caused her son's profound disabilities. No amount of tears, pleas, or denunciations could possibly restore Oliver's capabilities. But neither can I accept that, as the Dutch priest Henri J. M. Nouwen writes in the introduction, "these people [like Oliver] are God's messengers, they are the divine instruments of God's healing presence, they are the ones who bring truth to a society full of lies, light into the darkness and life into a death-oriented world."[11] I can't understand how a just God would deliberately create an empty shell like Oliver, or why He would deny an innocent child access to all the beauty and magic He allegedly created.

I'm not the first one to raise this objection, which is as old as the Bible itself and was most famously articulated by Rabbi Harold Kushner in his 1981 bestseller, *When Bad Things Happen to Good People*: "I am offended by those who suggest that God creates retarded children so that those around them will learn compassion and gratitude," he writes. "Why should God distort someone else's life to such a degree in order to enhance my spiritual sensitivity?" Kushner's solution is to strip God of his omnipotence, to argue that God "is limited in what He can do by laws of nature and by the evolution of human nature and human moral freedom." So Kushner's God "does not cause the bad things that happen to us," but, like a very human parent, "stands ready to help . . . us cope with our tragedies."[12]

Most believers reject this theory. "He is the Creator. He made every neuron, every combination of DNA, and every cell," insists Kelly Langston. "God's Word confirms this: 'Before I formed you in the womb I knew you' (Jeremiah 1:5)."[13] Other writers quote the book of Exodus, when God responds to Moses's protest that he is too "slow of speech" to advocate for the release of the Jewish people, "'Who gives man speech? Who makes him dumb or deaf, seeing or blind? Is it not I, the Lord?' (Exodus 4.11)."[14] The problem is not with God, but with mortal critics like Kushner. The theologian Douglas Blount argues, "We should expect *not* to understand God's reasons for acting as he does. . . . Thinking oneself capable of discerning God's reasons for acting as he does thus involves the stuff of which folly is made, namely, hubris."[15] These writers take the long view on justice, reminding us, as Langston does, "In the brilliant glory of God's eternity, there will be no trace—not the slightest breath—of autism. On that day, Alec will be healed, and not just partially—completely and forever healed."[16]

Ultimately, neither of these theories is particularly satisfying. I am sympathetic to Kushner's claim that he "can worship a God who hates suffering but cannot eliminate it more easily than I can worship a God who chooses to make children suffer and die, for whatever exalted reason."[17] But there's little solace in a God who can do nothing more than stand by wringing his hands at all the tragedy in the world. I might as well worship my eighty-nine-year-old father-in-law, whose parting words are always, "If everything goes right, I'll see you next Friday."

Honestly, I prefer the theology of Elon Musk, who believes we are all just characters in a computer simulation.[18] At least then Jonah's extreme impairments, the unfathomable fear of the Sandy Hook first graders, the Syrian kids gassed by their own government—none of that suffering would be real, only teaching modules designed to make me a better cyborg.

AND YET . . . EVEN as I refused to accept either the Old Testament God, who was so preoccupied with the smallest and most picayune details of religious practice that he immolated two priests (beloved sons of Moses's brother, Aaron) simply for offering the wrong kind of incense, or the New Testament version, who allows human suffering to enhance his own glory, I still couldn't completely let go of the idea of Jonah becoming a bar mitzvah. I'm not sure why. Of all the dreams for my son I'd already relinquished—college, career, marriage, children—this one seemed so minor in comparison, especially given my own tepid commitment to Judaism. I had never attended religious school myself, or celebrated my own bat mitzvah. Before my wedding, I had to persuade the rabbi that Andy wasn't marrying a *shiksa*, since I could neither read Hebrew nor recite even the most common prayers. Since then, I had raised my level of observance to match Andy's, but there was nothing particularly spiritual about it. I daydreamed through Rosh Hasha-nah services and suffered interminable Yom Kippur fasts. I duti-fully signed up our four younger kids for Sunday school when they entered first grade, but to a child they all hated it. (When Erika was about seven, she announced, "Hebrew school is pluck!" I asked her what she meant, and she confessed, "I'm using that word because it rhymes with another word that I'm not supposed to say that means bad." It was all I could do to stay composed as I asked my cherub, my innocent, insulated, copper-curled angel, "What word?" She eyed me for a moment, reluctant to say some-thing that might get her in trouble, then finally whispered, to my tremendous relief: "Yuck.") For me, being Jewish was like being American: it obviously defined me in important ways, but I rarely engaged with it directly.

Maybe a bar mitzvah was so appealing because it was the one completely typical rite of passage Jonah could experience. Once his aggressive and self-injurious behaviors were medically stabilized (at age eleven), I had no doubt he could learn to read Hebrew and participate in an adapted service. Jonah was hyperlexic as a child, intuiting how to read and write before he could talk. Although his comprehension skills remain extremely basic, he wouldn't need them for this endeavor—nobody did. Our synagogue, like many affiliated with the Reform movement, taught students to read He-brew but not to understand it. While I suspected it was exactly this endless, empty recitation that made Hebrew school so "pluck," at least it put Jonah and all the other bar and bat mitzvah candidates in the same liturgical boat. Perhaps it even gave Jonah a slight ad-vantage. Decoding lines of essentially meaningless text was right in his wheelhouse.

Despite my confidence in Jonah's ability to learn to read Hebrew, his thirteenth birthday came and went without any instruction.

I was paralyzed with indecision. For so long, his violent behaviors had precluded his participation in most activities. By the time he was nine, only Andy could manage the rages that erupted frequently and unpredictably, even at Jonah's favorite places: McDonald's, Costco, the beach and the zoo and the amusement park. Family outings were infrequent, carefully planned affairs. More often, we split up. I would take the four younger kids to the movies or the science museum or the paint-your-own pottery studio, and Andy would take Jonah shopping. Typically they would hit at least two big-box stores and one supermarket every weekend. I still don't know how Andy managed to keep Jonah close while wrangling an overflowing cart and checking every item off our endless lists. Only twice in all those years did he come home with an enormous sheet cake because Jonah bolted across the store to swipe a fingerful of frosting before Andy could stop him.

When Jonah's behaviors finally subsided, I couldn't wait to reunite my family. And we did. We finally took Jonah to my aunt's Hanukkah party and to our friends' annual summer barbecue bash. We took him to the pumpkin patch and to the fancy new playground his siblings always clamored to visit. We even went to Disney World.

It wasn't long before a new question emerged: Just because Jonah *could* do something, did that mean he *should*? When prompted, he would pick apples, bowl, or climb up a rock wall. But he didn't enjoy these activities. ("No apples," he would say. "No bowling." And we would say, with great enthusiasm, "Apples ONE more time!" which amused him for thirty seconds, at which point he would say again, "No apples.") Not only did Jonah not enjoy these outings, but they were stressful to manage. Without his structured routine, Jonah perseverated on food, often grabbing treats (or trying to) from other people. There were also legitimate safety concerns. From the time he was small, Jonah—like more than half of autistic children, according to recent studies—has been a wanderer. At home, we could relax, since we had long ago found all points of egress and sealed them off with coded bolts and key locks, but everywhere else Jonah required eyeballs on him every moment. Andy and I would trade off: one of us would join the other kids, or catch up with relatives at a family party, and the other would follow Jonah as he restlessly wandered from room to room, mostly watching *Sesame Street* videos on his iPad but occasionally and unpredictably dashing toward the food, or the door. After enough of these exhausting excursions, we decided that, as thrilled as we were that Jonah's behavior had stabilized sufficiently for him to be included with no meltdowns, we needed a new calculus: one that considered Jonah's interest, alternative activities he might prefer, and the impact taking him would have on the rest of the family.

Clearly, by any reasonable application of this formula, Hebrew school should have been categorically rejected. It's true that the rest of us would be minimally affected, since I would have to outsource this project, but I was certain both that Jonah would not enjoy his lessons and that there were a million better things he could do with the hundreds of hours they would occupy. Jonah couldn't cross the street safely. He couldn't answer open-ended questions like "How was your day?" He couldn't name the president, tell you what the president does, or understand the concepts, such as government and nation, one might use to explain it to him. Maybe the degree of his cognitive impairments meant he would never learn. But wasn't it more worthwhile to try than to teach him an incomprehensible language he would never use after showcasing his skill at a bar mitzvah service that would remain as fundamentally inaccessible to him as a trick performed by a trained animal—and that's where I cut myself off, every time. But never quickly enough to stop the flood of guilt and grief that hit so hard I physically recoiled, shaking my head, clenching my eyes closed. How could I, even in the darkest and most uncontrollable corners of my mind, compare my own son to a dog or horse being put through his paces in return for praise and snacks? I couldn't, I shouldn't, so I shoved it all down like the puppet in the jack-in-the-box and slammed the lid. I wouldn't even consider the possibility of Jonah's religious education again for months afterward.

And yet . . . I couldn't let it go. I thought I had, many times, but it always came back.

WE DECIDED TO start slow. Erika's bat mitzvah was scheduled for September 2014, and as it approached I wondered what part Jonah should play. He would never be able to sit through the entire two-hour service, but he could certainly come in for a few minutes: to march with the Torah around the synagogue, to read an English translation, to say a prayer. I decided that I wanted Jonah to join Andy and me in an *aliyah*, which is the blessing that is recited before reading the Torah.

Jonah certainly could have read an English transliteration. Many neurotypical people shamelessly take this shortcut, but I didn't even consider it. There was a limit to what I would cede to autism. Sometimes I surprised even myself at where I drew the line: holiday cards, for instance. For many years, I spent more time agonizing over the conception and execution of our annual holiday card than I did decorating, cooking, or picking out gifts. The picture had to be perfect: one photo, with all five kids looking great. This was extraordinarily difficult, since the rages Jonah suffered when he was younger made photo shoots frustrating and unpredictable. But I steadfastly refused the alternative, which was to use templates available on websites like Shutterfly and just drag and drop five separate pictures of my kids (even though many of my friends did just that, because whether your children are autistic or not it's a challenge to take one photo in which everyone looks good, particularly when toddlers are involved). Getting this one fabulous photo took on massive symbolism for me. We couldn't take exotic vacations like many of my friends did over the break; we couldn't even go, together as a family, to parties or to the movies for the traditional "Jewish Christmas." So the card became the one small corner I staked out of the holiday landscape, the one completely typical ritual in which all my kids could participate, and I would not be moved off it.

There were other factors involved in my decision to teach Jonah enough Hebrew to read the aliyah. Primarily, I wanted to test my theory that he would pick it up fairly easily. Jonah was fifteen, but I still hadn't given up the idea that he would have his own bar mitzvah. Now my hope was that one day the two of us could celebrate a joint *b'nai mitzvah*—*b'nai* being the plural of *bar* and *bat*. I had always planned on going through it, since it seemed hypocritical to subject the kids to a Hebrew education I didn't consider important enough to pursue for myself. I had even started attending a language class: no transliteration for me either.

We hired a tutor to come to the house once a week. Barbara was a retired special education teacher who came highly recommended. I don't think she had ever worked with anyone as severely affected as Jonah, but she wasn't intimidated. She showed up with flashcards, puzzles, a whiteboard—whatever she thought might hold his attention. And jellybeans, to reward him after a successful activity. It didn't bother me as much as I thought it would. Restricted interests are one of the core symptoms of autism. Not much motivates Jonah besides his iPad and food. Most of the skills he learned in school—from rolling silverware for a retirement community to using a debit card to walking on a treadmill—have been shaped with edible reinforcers.

Jonah spent most of Erika's bat mitzvah service in the empty social hall watching videos with an aide. One of the synagogue administrators slipped out to get him right before the Torah service, while Erika carried the heavy scrolls around the sanctuary and the rest of our family followed in a little processional, stopping every few feet to quickly embrace our guests and allow them to touch the Torah with their prayer shawls and books. I was hiccupping with the mostly unsuccessful effort of holding back sobs. It was an emotional day, for sure: I was proud of Erika, and overwhelmed at seeing so many people we loved—many of whom had traveled great distances to share the joyous day. But I was also unbearably anxious. I just wanted Jonah to do well. I wanted him to stand on the *bimah* with us and read the blessing like I had seen him do hundreds of times over the past year. We had prepared him for this moment as best we could, including taking him to the synagogue to practice in the empty sanctuary. But who knew how he would react now that the pews were filled? Many of our friends and extended family members had known Jonah his whole life. I knew they wouldn't judge if he suddenly lay down on the floor or began yelling or biting his hand in agitation. But that day I wanted them to be impressed by what Jonah could do, not by everything he couldn't.

And they were. Jonah said the entire aliyah—slowly, tunelessly, but he read the entire blessing. At the party, many people told me how moved they were by Jonah's participation. Later that week a friend emailed me a picture she had surreptitiously snapped with her phone, even though photography is expressly forbidden during the service: Jonah at the lectern, surrounded by me, Andy,

Erika, the rabbi, and the cantor. That blurry and pixilated image got its own page in Erika's bat mitzvah album, next to the beautifully composed work of our professional photographer.

After that, preparations for our b'nai mitzvah began in earnest. In addition to weekly sessions with Barbara, Jonah began attending a special-needs religious school at a different local synagogue. Every Sunday, he studied with his own private teacher, practicing Hebrew and working through very basic lessons about Jewish figures, holidays, and rituals. He watched cartoons about Joseph and his brothers, colored pictures of fruit to hang in the *sukkah*, and read short passages with titles like "What Is a Blessing?" I was never sure what, if anything, Jonah took away from these activities. All I can say for certain is that for the first year I refused to leave the synagogue during his three-hour classes, afraid the teacher would need my help if Jonah became agitated or refused to participate, but he never did.

What if religion weren't really about God? What if all those elements that make it incomprehensible to Jonah—from the commandments to the cosmology—are merely adornments, secondary to a vital purpose that moves each and every one of us?

Émile Durkheim was a French sociologist working at the beginning of the twentieth century who set out to uncover the common base underlying all religions. He immediately discarded belief in God, since several major religions—including Buddhism and Jainism—are essentially atheistic. Using the simple, totemic systems of aboriginal tribes as case studies, Durkheim concluded that religion is, first and foremost, the symbolic representation of society. Its primary purpose is not, he argued, to explain natural phenomena like death or the sun, but to connect us to our community. As the scholar Mark Cladis explained in his introduction to Durkheim's 1912 book *The Elementary Forms of Religious Life*, "A society whose members were consumed by narrow self-interest and mundane activities would eventually disintegrate.... Religion, in contrast, links individuals to each other and to society by animating their lives with the sacred: powerful symbols—including 'secular' ones—that make and remake society's collective existence.... In the absence of common, sacred aims, human flourishing cannot take place."[19]

I didn't discover Durkheim until after our b'nai mitzvah, but when I did his book finally answered the question that had nagged at me throughout the preparations and all the years I had spent agonizing over it: Why did I want this so badly? Honestly, I thought I would never know. I guess I attributed that decision to the same incoherent yet strangely persistent desires that drove me to have five kids, to apply to graduate school at the age of forty-six, and to eat myself sick, many times, on chocolate frosting straight out of the tub.

Arguably, I should have figured this one out on my own. When I used to imagine our b'nai mitzvah, I didn't picture Jonah reciting the *motze* over a golden braid of challah, or leading the congregation in the lovely and reverent *sh'ma*—although he did say both these prayers during the service. Instead, I envisioned all the aides and teachers who had loved Jonah since he was in kindergarten coming back to celebrate with us. I wondered how Jonah would react to such a *This Is Your Life* moment: Would he bounce up and down and clap? Say their names? Step down from the bimah for a closer look? (During one follow-up visit to the hospital where Jonah was inpatient for most of his tenth year, we had lunch with a few members of his old care team. Although it hadn't been long since his discharge, one of his favorite aides had cut her hair short. Jonah went up to give her a hug, but paused to read her name off her identification badge, just to make sure.) I knew he remembered them all—once in a while even the names of people we hadn't seen in a decade popped up in Jonah's running monologue. I couldn't guess what he would think about them all suddenly showing up in one place. But I was certain there would be smiles, embraces, exclamations over how tall and handsome he was.

If these reunion fantasies weren't enough to convince me that our b'nai mitzvah was most importantly, for me, a community-building exercise—one that would, as Durkheim wrote of all religious ceremonies, "bring individuals together . . . increase contacts between them, and . . . make those contacts more intimate"[20]— I might have noticed that other parents of severely autistic kids I turned to for guidance echoed startlingly similar sentiments. When I asked Debbie, a Facebook friend, why she and her husband decided to teach her ten-year-old stepson, Scott, to take first communion, she told me that her husband "wanted to make his father happy and his family happy." Their church did not welcome Scott into the religious school because of his behaviors, so Debbie and her husband tried to prepare him by reading picture books and attempting to do exercises from a workbook the church sent home. Although Scott had little tolerance for the worksheets, he did learn how to cross himself and performed perfectly at the ceremony. "You know, sometimes our kids have these times when they rise to the occasion, and this was one of those days," Debbie told me. "I think Scott knew how important it was, and held it together. It's not usual for him to behave appropriately, it was like a little miracle."[21] Afterwards, the entire family celebrated with a party in the private room of a restaurant.

The writer and autism advocate Susan Senator held a bar mitzvah for her autistic son, Nat, now twenty-six, but not for either of his younger brothers—so she clearly wasn't motivated by religious reasons. "He wasn't going to have much celebration in his life," Susan said. "I knew there'd be no middle school graduation or anything like that, so we wanted something special for him." She rented a room in a fancy hotel, and invited sixty people—family, friends, former teachers, and staff. "I was so proud of him," Susan remembered. "He wore my father's *tallis* [prayer shawl] from his bar mitzvah. Both sides of our family were there. Nat was really on, really focused, and looks beautiful in all the pictures, really aware. The whole day I was floating on a cloud, it was such a triumph."[22]

Maybe I did know. Traditionally, bar and bat mitzvah candidates write a *d'var Torah*—an analysis of their Torah portion—and read it to the congregation during the service. This is how mine ended:

> Preparing Jonah to become a bar mitzvah took a team of religious leaders and educators from two local synagogues, as well as years of private tutoring, and every single person involved in this process was not only patient, flexible, and encouraging, but they all embraced Jonah as an important and valued member of the Jewish community. And this emphasis on inclusion and support is prioritized in the Torah, even if it's not explicitly applied to the disabled. In fact, it happens to be the subject of my *parashah*, or Torah portion. It comes from the book of Deuteronomy, in which Moses gives the Israelites a lengthy and quite particular list of instructions on how to live a holy life. This week's *parashah* contains several commands concerning the care of the most vulnerable; Moses instructs the Jewish people, "When you reap the harvest in your field and overlook a sheaf in the field, do not turn back to get it; it shall go to the stranger, the fatherless, and the widow." He emphasizes that we must care for one another, even at great inconvenience. If we find something that has been lost, we must return it to its rightful owner, and if we encounter a "fellow's ass or ox fallen on the road"—an admittedly unlikely event, nowadays—we "must help him raise it." The command that sums up these directions, "You must not remain indifferent," is nothing less than "the ethical

demand of Torah," according to the Jewish scholar Harvey J. Fields, who adds, "Indifference is intolerable. Responsible caring is at the heart of Jewish ethics."

The Old Testament was written almost 3,500 years ago. Of course it contains artifacts of that culture that make us uncomfortable—not just concerning the disabled, but also about women, homosexuals, and slaves. But that mandate, "You must not remain indifferent," is just as powerful today as the day it was written. And whether you knew about it or not, it drives every person in this room. At some point in the last decade, Jonah needed you, and you were there for him. He screamed and hit and kicked, and it would have been so easy and so understandable for those of you who worked with him during those years to walk away, but you all stayed—and not only did you stay, you loved him anyway. We would never have gotten to this point—where Jonah is stable, and happy, and successful in school and I am writing and advocating for other families who almost always are not nearly as lucky as mine—without your effort and commitment. So, while today we are officially celebrating Jonah's and my b'nai mitzvah, what I am celebrating most of all is the overwhelming support—the opposite of indifference, if you will—that lifted us out of some incredibly dark days and continues to nurture and inspire both me and Jonah, even if he may seem more focused on the platters of pretzels and cinnamon rolls at the party than on catching up. Words cannot describe how grateful I am to have had you in our lives, but since that's all I've got: thank you.

"Not only did you stay, you loved him anyway." For Durkheim, everything in the world could be divided into two categories, the sacred and the profane. That was the most sacred moment of my entire life.

I WISH I COULD say that our b'nai mitzvah was also a special day for Jonah. But even though his medical regimen keeps him mostly stable, some days he's more agitated than others. I knew before we left the house this was one of those days. Jonah absolutely refused to wear the collared shirt I picked out for him. "No button," he insisted over and over, trying to grab it out of my hand—to rip it, or shove it in his trash can.

"OK," I said, slipping it back on the hanger. "No button." I had anticipated Jonah might reject the collared shirt—although he wears one at a work site he goes to during the school day, he's never really liked them—and had also purchased a new crewneck shirt that was the same burgundy as my dress. He accepted the new shirt, but his mood didn't particularly improve.

We arrived at the synagogue a few minutes before the one-thirty service, and my composure lasted about as long as it took to walk from the car to the chapel. I started crying as soon as I saw Jen, who had worked for us until she graduated from Villanova in 2009. She came to us as a perky sorority sister who answered an ad we posted at the university looking for aides—an English major who had no experience working with autistic kids. But Jonah responded right away to her enthusiasm. We used to joke about his taste in women, because we had a series of pretty, young aides—hired by the county or the school district, or recruited by us from local colleges or the special-needs camp Jonah attended when summer school wasn't in session—and Jonah loved them all. So many of them came back for the b'nai mitzvah: Melissa, Rael, Amanda, even Ashley, who had flown in from Seattle, where she has since relocated, because she didn't want to miss it.

There were others, also: most of Jonah's team of kindergarten teachers came, as well as more recent members of our home team: Ky, Shaneen, Lora. The doctors who had successfully treated him drove from New York and Maryland. As each new person walked in, I watched Jonah, hoping for some kind of reaction, and when there was none, I coaxed him: "Jonah, look, it's Miss Elliott! Say hi to Miss Elliott!" For her, the old teacher he had never completely stopped asking for, he did seem to momentarily brighten. But then it passed; he just repeated, "Say hi to Miss Elliott," and resumed repeating the title of the *Sesame Street* DVD he had been perseverating on all morning: "*HVN Flowers, Bananas and More* DVD Sony Wonder."

"First Hebrew, then *Flowers, Bananas and More*," I said.

"DVD Sony Wonder," he added.

"DVD Sony Wonder," I corrected. "Jonah, don't you want to say hi to Mrs. Gaspar?" Or Sam or Maria or Aunt Rita?

"*HVN Flowers, Bananas and More* DVD Sony Wonder." And so on.

Jonah actually did a fantastic job with his part of the service. He earned a laugh from the audience when he prematurely recited the aliyah, interrupting the cantor as she explained the prayer to the mostly non-Jewish crowd, and another when he drained the entire goblet of grape juice after saying the *kiddush*. But in between, he kept trying to leave. He tugged at my arm to get me to come with him. In his most agitated moments, he bit his hand and yelled. Was he overwhelmed by all the people? Maybe, although the fact that he had been irritable all day suggested that this mood, like so many of his, was internally driven. It was impossible to know.

Jonah did dive into the food we served at the party we held at our house afterwards. We had all his favorites: hamburgers, salt-and-vinegar potato chips, soft pretzels with cheddar cheese dip. He ate as much as he wanted—but seriously, without engaging with anyone sitting around him. When he was full, he wandered around the party, holding his iPad, and insisting, "*HVN Flowers, Bananas and More* DVD Sony Wonder." Even the much anticipated (by everyone else in the family) arrival of Nick, one of Jonah's most beloved aides, didn't provoke a smile. Nick must have spent hundreds of hours drawing for Jonah during the two years he worked for us; of all our aides, he was the most accomplished artist, mastering even Barney, a character I still can't do well. Now, he's the father of infant twin girls, who we fussed over while Jonah cycled from me to Andy to our nanny, Marina: "*HVN Flowers, Bananas and More DVD Sony Wonder.*"

Finally, after dessert had been served and the guests had begun to leave, I told Marina she could take Jonah to Barnes and Noble, since he wanted to go so badly. "It's his day," I told myself, "he should do what he wants." And perhaps nothing better illustrates the heartbreaking frustration of severe autism than this: after asking for it all day, Jonah found the DVD he wanted at the bookstore, examined it, then put it back in the bin and walked out empty-handed.

But none of this means the b'nai mitzvah was a failure. Émile Durkheim writes, "Acts of worship, whatever they might be, are not futile or meaningless gestures. By seeming to strengthen the ties between the worshipper and his god, they really strengthen the ties that bind the individual to society."[23] And who needs community more than families like mine, like Debbie's, like Susan's? Nothing is more isolating than severe autism. We've been phenomenally lucky to have the support we've had, but that is in no way typical. Many parents are frequently stuck at home, because their kids can neither be safely taken out nor left with a babysitter. They may not feel comfortable inviting guests to goggle at their patched walls and stained carpets, or they may just be too exhausted from running a behavior plan until their kids go to bed— *if* they go to bed—to entertain. And let's face it, we can become pretty prickly—just try asking us if we've heard about the kid who was cured by watching Disney movies. Inevitably, for far too many families, the invitations just stop coming.

Everyone needs, and everyone deserves, the feeling of connection I had as I stood in front of that chapel. Maybe Jonah didn't feel it; maybe he did and didn't show it. Either way, it doesn't end there. I made an album that we keep in Jonah's room: pictures of the service and the party, all the people who were important in his life and wanted him to know that he was still important in theirs. I've read it with him; right now he doesn't seem too interested. By the time he picks it up on his own, he might very well have forgotten all the Hebrew he ever learned. But each time he looks at it, he will know: he is not, and has never been, alone.

9

Baseline

In the video, Jonah is rolling on the floor, yelling and crying. At the left edge of the screen is a sneaker he kicked off; at the right are the bare arms of two school aides, trying to block my son from banging his head against the furniture. At times he moves his hand to his face to suck his thumb, as if he's trying to calm himself; at others he bites so hard it's astonishing there's no blood. When he starts to hit his head, staff step in to block the punches. In the background, over the sound of Jonah's screams and his fist pounding the wall—shockingly loud, as if it were made of metal— I hear voices: an aide, asking if he wants to "do a fun list," one of his favorite leisure activities; another offering a blanket; the school psychologist, wondering if hot or cold compresses might soothe him; the director, noting that "he's never been like this"—which was, of course, why they were recording this behavior, which lasted the entire day: November 14, 2017.

Actually, Jonah has been like this countless times, or even worse—just not since he moved to his current school in 2013. Watching the video, I couldn't help marveling that, as agitated as he was, he never attacked anyone—the main difference between this episode and the rages he used to suffer daily, during which he would launch himself at us, his teachers, and his aides. When

I try to remember what it was like to fight with my son, I see only hands: one wrapped over Jonah's fist, another under his jaw to keep him from biting, another untangling my hair from his fingers, one intercepting before he could yank another necklace off my neck—because that's what it was, a blur of hands. I never had enough hands.

We lived like that for the better part of a decade, until electroconvulsive therapy (ECT) stabilized Jonah's rapid-cycling bipolar disorder in 2010—after exhaustive medication trials, elaborate behavior plans, even a ten-month hospitalization all failed.[1] Nine years later, Jonah still gets ECT three times a month. Typically, his behavior remains consistent. Occasionally, toward the end of the treatment interval, he experiences mild episodes of agitation with no obvious environmental triggers. Jonah's meltdown—the worst we had seen in years—happened on the day before ECT.

The next day, Jonah went to school after his morning appointment, just like he always does, the grogginess induced by both the seizure and the anesthesia wearing off in the car during the forty-minute ride. After lunch, I received a text from the director: "Back to baseline today . . . he is doing well."

LATER, THIS STRUCK me as an odd choice of words. I had always understood "baseline"—at least in medical contexts—to refer to an original, predisease state. Treatments were therapeutic to the extent they restored optimal, baseline functioning.

But what if the original state was itself pathological? Jonah in his baseline, pre-ECT condition was ferocious in his rage. I could just barely fend him off when he was eleven years old; now, at twenty, he has five inches and fifty pounds on me. It should be unsettling, I suppose, to think that in his natural state my son would be a legitimate threat to kill me. But we've been living with necessary and transformative psychiatric intervention for so long—not just with Jonah, but with my middle daughter Hilary, now sixteen, who has been taking stimulants for ADHD since she was in third grade—that what's actually been unsettled is any privilege I ever assigned to the natural in the first place.

I would hardly call mine a consensus position. Opponents of medicating children are fierce and pervasive—in books with ominous titles like *The Silenced Child* and *Suffer the Children*, as well as in countless articles featured on well-respected platforms. On the *Psychology Today* website, Robert Berezin lamented, "If they're active give them amphetamines; if they're moody give them Prozac; for fears, give them benzodiazepines; and while we're at it, let's give them antipsychotics, or Lithium and other mood stabilizing drugs. What in the world are we doing?"[2] Hanif Kureishi, writing in the *New York Times*, was more graphic: "Ritalin and other forms of enforcement and psychological policing are the contemporary equivalent of the old practice of tying up children's hands in bed, so they won't touch their genitals."[3]

Many of these opponents simply don't believe in ADHD or other psychiatric diagnoses given to children. Marilyn Wedge, the author of *Suffer the Children*, defends intervention for adults but argues, "There is no indication at all that either the diagnoses or treatments that work for adults apply to kids."[4] In *The Silenced Child*, Claudia Gold maintains that "diagnostic labels and psychiatric drugs are symptoms of a cultural shift away from valuing human relationships."[5] The title of Berezin's post nicely sums up this position: "No, There Is No Such Thing as ADHD."

The persistence of this delusion is mildly distressing, but I don't spend too much time thinking about it. It's impossible to debate with those so disconnected from reality that they honestly believe, as Gold argues, "There is no 'truth' for the diagnosis of autism or, for that matter, any other DSM-defined 'mental disorders,' all of which are based on subjective assessments of behavior or 'symptoms.'"[6] While there is admittedly no blood test or simple genetic marker for autism, ADHD, schizophrenia, or mood disorders, to bracket their symptoms with disdainful airquotes is to dismiss, for example, the hallucinations that caused the writer Michael Schofield's schizophrenic daughter, January, to attack her parents, her baby brother, and the family dog, as well as the crippling paranoia that confined a bipolar teenage boy I know to his home, cowering in fear that the Burger King mascot would come rape him.[7] Would Gold actually suggest that Jonah—with his minimal language, his perseverative behaviors, his complete disinterest in peers, and his history of purposeless rages—doesn't "truly" have autism? It's impossible to imagine that, confronted with these profoundly debilitated children, Gold would blame, as she does in her book, "the lack of opportunity for calm reflection."[8]

ADHD is harder to defend by this reasoning, as the associated problems and behaviors—including distractibility, reactivity, and disorganization—are far less disturbing, and individually may also occur in typical children. Berezin, for example, argues that kids with ADHD are actually just "stereotypical boys" whose parents "are giving insufficient loving attention to the child."[9]

This odd logic—rejecting ADHD on the one hand while blaming parents for this supposedly fictional diagnosis on the other—is surprisingly, and sadly, common. It evokes Bruno Bettelheim's long discredited "refrigerator mother" theory of autism etiology, which states that "the precipitating factor in infantile autism is the parent's wish that his child should not exist."[10] Marilyn Wedge agrees that "jumpiness" and other symptoms are "evidence of something wrong in the family," while Francis Fukuyama—a political scientist with absolutely no medical training whatsoever—self-righteously condemns "parents and teachers who do not want to spend the time and energy necessary to discipline, divert, entertain, or train difficult children the old-fashioned way" for "taking a medical shortcut."[11]

Importantly, however, the vast majority of physicians and researchers reject this recasting of ADHD as "a conflict between today's Huckleberry Finns and their caregivers."[12] In 2002, over eighty scientists from five continents signed the "International Consensus Statement on ADHD," which included more than five hundred citations from researchers all over the world recognizing the legitimacy of this disorder. The authors offer this definition of a "valid medical or psychiatric disorder": "there must be scientifically established evidence that those suffering the condition have a serious deficiency in or failure of a physical or psychological mechanism that is universal to humans. . . . And there must be equally incontrovertible scientific evidence that this serious deficiency leads to harm to the individual." ADHD clearly meets these criteria. The signers go on to list some of the more notable consequences: "sufferers are far more likely than normal people to drop out of school (32–40%) . . . to have few or no friends (50–70%), to underperform at work (70–80%), to engage in antisocial activities (40–50%) . . . and in hundreds of other ways mismanage and endanger their lives."[13] In short, rejecting the validity of ADHD involves embracing a worldwide conspiracy of internationally renowned scientists, universities, and hospitals that makes the most gonzo theories about Roswell and the JFK assassination look like tooth-fairy tales. Perhaps that's why even a critic like Alan Schwarz opens *ADHD Nation*, his investigation into misdiagnosis and overmedication, with this assertion: "Attention deficit hyperactivity disorder is real."[14]

While I find the complete deniers easy to ignore, there is a concern that I find harder to dismiss: whether psychiatric interventions fundamentally alter our personalities, our identities, our sense of self. That's what Claudia Gold is getting at when she claims that psychotropic medication "essentially puts a muzzle on the child"; Peter Breggin describes this as a "chemical lobotomy."[15] This is scary stuff, evoking the famous story of Phineas Gage, who in 1848 suffered a traumatic brain injury when a tamping iron speared his skull following a railroad explosion. Prior to the accident, Gage had been considered smart, hard-working, responsible, and kind. After he miraculously recovered, however, he was markedly different: prone to profanity, impatient, impulsive, unreliable. When my four younger children were each in fifth grade, they participated in a debate one of the teachers organizes every year: Did Phineas Gage die that day? (The kids, incidentally, preferred to be on the negative side, so they could make the obvious technical argument: Gage's heart did not stop beating—in fact, shockingly, he never even lost consciousness—so, de facto, he didn't die. Fifth graders are not particularly prone to existential angst.)

I, however, am not so sure. More recently, Jason Padgett writes about the brain injury that had the opposite effect on him than it had on Gage. Instead of a host of negative effects, Padgett reports that the violent mugging he suffered in 2002 turned him into a mathematical genius. Thirty-one at the time, he had been a slacker, a college drop-out who worked in his father's furniture stores. Since then, he sees the world geometrically: fractals in the swirl of cream in his coffee, the Pythagorean theorem in the leaves of trees, pi in the "half-dome curvature of the sky." His astonishing gift, as well as his newfound ability to capture these visions in precise mathematical drawings—lattices based on Planck lengths and radiating circles based on prime numbers—led to a diagnosis of acquired savant syndrome. Instead of selling futons, he is now studying to be a number theorist. Did Jason Padgett die after his attack? In his memoir, he writes, "I knew I had a life before this one—a full and happy one in its crazy way—but I was no longer that man."[16]

Fictional examples provide even less ambiguous cases—such as the 1991 movie *Regarding Henry*, in which Harrison Ford plays an unscrupulous, narcissistic, philandering attorney who, after being shot during a robbery, is utterly transformed into a gentle, rather simple man with completely different career, food, clothing, and even hairstyle preferences. Or Lisa Genova's 2007 novel *Still Alice*, whose protagonist starts off a Harvard professor and ends with Alzheimer's disease so advanced she doesn't know her husband or her children. Certainly, I believe that whatever was "Henry," whatever was "Alice"—despite any fifth graders that might insist otherwise—was dead. So I obviously also think that the self enjoys only so much latitude before it becomes other. Was memory loss the crucial factor? Henry and Alice both became almost completely amnesiac. But, while memories are doubtlessly important, different scenes stick with me from those stories: Henry spontaneously buying a puppy; Alice placidly licking an ice cream cone next to the Charles River, unconcerned that she no longer remembers the university where she used to work.[17] No, memory loss isn't everything, or even the most critical thing.

Maybe it's the violence of the rupture, the unnatural pace of change. If Henry and Alice were ninety years old, we would expect them to be slower, softer, more insular in their concerns. And then I think about how quickly Jonah transformed, after three weeks of ECT, from a child who came after us multiple times a day to one who didn't rage at all, and I appreciate that it is not an absurd question, whether or not he is still the same.

BEFORE ASSESSING HOW much their medical interventions have changed Jonah and Hilary, it's worth asking what *Jonah* and *Hilary* even mean. Antipsychiatric rhetoric implies there is a stable, coherent self that is threatened by medication or ECT—an idea that reflects the mind-body dualism first articulated by René Descartes in the seventeenth century. Three hundred years later, the British philosopher Gilbert Ryle dubbed this theory "the Ghost in the Machine."[18] Although Ryle was speaking disparagingly, this metaphor pretty accurately reflects typical human phenomenology. It does feel like there's something in there, driving the proverbial bus. At least something ephemeral, like a ghost, is marginally less absurd than a tiny homunculus.

But neuroscientists have shown that this feeling of subjectivity is largely an illusion. The psychological researcher Michael Gazzaniga explains, "The view in neuroscience today is that consciousness does not constitute a single, generalized process . . . [but] a multitude of widely distributed specialized systems and disunited processes." The unity we feel is an illusion generated by an "interpreter module" whose job is to "generate explanations about our perceptions, memories, and actions and the relationships among them."[19]

Gazzaniga cites fascinating examples of how the interpreter module can be fooled, nicely exposing its need to provide a consistent, ongoing narrative. Many of these come from studies done on patients whose corpora callosa—the nerve fibers connecting the left and right hemispheres of the brain—have been cut, typically to treat intractable epilepsy. The interpreter module is on the left side of the brain, so activity on the right side is inaccessible to the patients' interpreters. That doesn't stop them from concocting explanations, however. One patient's right hemisphere was shown a fire safety video in which a man is pushed into a fire. Although the patient could not describe what she had seen beyond "'just a white flash,'" she needed a reason to explain why she suddenly felt so anxious. First she blamed the room, then she decided she was scared of Gazzaniga himself.[20]

Gazzaniga also suggests that phobias can result from creative storytelling from our interpreter modules. He notes that spontaneous cerebral activity can cause symptoms such as sweating and elevated heart rate that the interpreter will be desperate to explain. "Most people's interpretive system would take cues from their own unique past and present psychological history and the current environmental cues to come up with an explanation," he writes. "I must be scared, and what can be scaring me must be . . . [looks around and sees a dog] a dog! I am scared of dogs!"[21]

The Israeli historian Yuval Noah Harari agrees with Gazzaniga, although he uses different terminology: "We identify with the inner system that takes the crazy chaos of life and spins out of it seemingly logical and consistent yarns."[22] It's important to reiterate, however, that this interpreter module is not just another word for the self. Rather, its job is to create the illusion of coherence from a consciousness that is actually "engendered by multiple modules, each of which has specialized capacities . . . [and] is distributed everywhere across the brain."[23] As Harari summarizes, "The single authentic self is as real as the eternal soul, Santa Claus and the Easter Bunny."[24]

It's somewhat unmooring, to read a line like that. But at the same time, I found it unsurprising—kind of like the completely unexpected twist in a great novel that, in retrospect, was the only way the plot could have unfolded. I remember nothing about being five years old, and I suspect, were I magically transported into my kindergarten brain, I would find it very foreign. I don't even feel particularly connected to my college-age self. The multiplicity that Gazzaniga describes makes sense to me. It recognizes how many different parts contribute to our experience of the self: evolutionary inheritance, genetic predisposition, environmental influence. It acknowledges the importance of memories, relationships, skills, and preferences while also celebrating the flexibility to absorb significant changes in any of these elements. After all, when I think about Jonah's and Hilary's most defining characteristics—Jonah's love of *Sesame Street* and Hilary's of Dungeons and Dragons; Jonah's obsession with ketchup and Hilary's with reading; Jonah's need to spin and Hilary's to spend time alone daydreaming—I understand that, ten years from now, maybe none of those will still apply, and yet I won't consider them completely different people.

If the self is so fluid, then what exactly is "muzzled" and "lobotomized" by psychotropic medication? Importantly, these descriptors were articulated by adults criticizing the medication of children, not the children themselves. When researchers finally asked them, in a 2012 British study, how their medication made them feel, over 90 percent of young subjects reported that their stimulants did not compromise their sense of authenticity. Rather, they appreciated "the potential for self-actualization via the development of self-control." Researcher Ilina Singh notes that claims suggesting "that children are 'stupefied' by Ritalin, or turned into mindless, obedient zombies, unfairly characterizes a majority of children's capacities for self-reflection and moral awareness while taking medication and disregards the high value children place on their capacity for moral agency, which many experience as being enabled by medication."[25]

I can't ask Jonah how he feels about his medical regimen, but after I read this study, I couldn't wait to ask Hilary the same questions posed to Singh's young subjects. I kind of knew what she would say on a general level, because I'd obviously been periodically checking in with her for the past seven years. Still, I was a little surprised—both by her excitement about our interview, and by how emphatic and articulate she was in her responses. Hilary told me that when she takes her medicine, "I feel like my conscious self—the person I want to be—is more in control." She said that she can tell when she's forgotten her morning dose: "I can't focus on anything. I get distracted by the snow falling outside, or that my hair is suddenly super interesting. I also get mood swings—I crack up at the slightest provocation, but if someone scolds me, I get really sad." When she said that I couldn't help remembering a phone call I got from her third-grade teacher after one especially chaotic morning when I had forgotten to give Hilary her stimulant. Miss Unger wanted to know, had anything changed? Hilary had spent the first part of the day immersed in a book rather than attending to the teacher, and when Miss Unger moved her to a spot at the front of the room to encourage more engagement, Hilary disassembled the model intended for a math lesson right under the teacher's nose. "Hilary's just not available for learning today," Miss Unger reported, diplomatically.

What I found most fascinating about my conversation with Hilary was her location of authenticity with her medicated self. She told me, "I feel great when I'm on [my stimulant] because when I'm not, I feel that my true self is blocked by a thousand layers of foam wall. It's like peeling back layers of red tape, there are fewer obstacles in the way."

Interestingly, it was exactly this sentiment—as expressed by adults who had been prescribed Prozac—that inspired the bestselling book *Listening to Prozac*. Peter Kramer quotes one patient who reports, "[It's] as if I had been in a drugged state all those years and now I am clearheaded." Another claims that "Prozac had let her personality emerge at last—she had not been alive before taking an antidepressant." These accounts forced Kramer to consider whether "medication somehow removed a false self and replaced it with a true one."[26]

These reports—from Hilary, from Singh, from Kramer—left me inspired, even liberated, by their redefinition of authenticity. Some of us, many of us, need help—for ADHD, autism, mood disorders, schizophrenia, anxiety. Some of us are prone to addiction, others to aggression. In his book *The Anatomy of Violence*, the psychologist Adrian Raine describes the physiological factors that predispose some individuals to criminal behavior, including enzyme deficiencies, neurotransmitter levels, metabolic rates, and anomalies in brain structure. He is a strong advocate for pharmaceutical intervention to decrease aggression in this population. Does minimizing or even eradicating a person's violent thoughts change him or her into a totally different person? Raine does not address this concern, because—echoing Harari and Gazzaniga—he also thinks the self is an illusion: "You want so desperately to believe that you determine things in your life, yet that belief has no true substance. It floats like a ghost in a mind machine forged by ancient evolutionary forces."[27]

Raine's murderers provide an important counternarrative to the "Huckleberry Finn" tale spun by critics of psychopharmacology. Those serial killers and bar-brawlers perfectly illustrate the misconception so frequently driving this debate, which the English philosopher G. E. Moore termed the "naturalistic fallacy" in 1903. He advised, "We must not, therefore, be frightened by the assertion that a thing is natural into the admission that it is good; good does not, by definition, mean anything that is natural; and it is therefore always an open question whether anything that is natural is good."[28]

Over a century later, this fallacy is still pervasive. Reflected in the critiques of ADHD naysayers like Robert Berezin, Claudia Gold, and Peter Breggin, it is perhaps most perfectly illustrated by Francis Fukuyama, who suggests that "ADHD isn't a disease at all but rather just the tail of the bell curve describing the distribution of perfectly normal behavior."[29] The same, after all, can be said about much pathology: diabetics reflect the tail of pancreatic functioning; the deaf inhabit the tail of auditory functioning; and the violent offenders featured in *The Anatomy of Violence* represent the tail of the bell curve describing the distribution of human aggression. Yet few people would argue that the unadulterated brains of Raine's subjects would not have benefitted from psychiatric interventions to make them less reactive or more empathetic. The question is not whether ADHD, autism, or aggression (or diabetes or cancer or depression) is *natural*. It's whether or not we can do better, when nature isn't enough.

This is not at all to suggest that today's ADHD children will grow into tomorrow's psychopaths. Rather, it's to point out that, instead of imagining rambunctious boys innocently tumbling over one another like puppies, we need to foreground the real struggles and suffering that precipitate psychiatric intervention. Having arrived at a point where Jonah no longer tries to rip my hair out and Hilary can weather minor injustices, like students cutting in front of her in the cafeteria, without completely losing her composure and alienating her peers with unwarranted hysterics, I've stopped caring about what is innate. And when I wonder about the self—because even though I rationally accept the neuroscientific rejection of this concept, as Michael Gazzaniga notes, it "is a powerful and overwhelming illusion that is almost impossible to shake"[30]—I don't think about uncovering a true or authentic self, theirs or mine. Instead, I focus on the hard work of constructing our very best selves. And I'm grateful to live in a time when we are no longer as constrained by our biology as we once were; when our baseline is not merely descriptive but potentially catalytic, a springboard to countless conceivable futures.

Notes

Preface

1 Joanne Kaufman, "Ransom-Note Ads about Children's Health Are Canceled," *New York Times*, December 20, 2007, https://www.nytimes.com/2007/12/20/business/media/20child.html.

2 "Frequently Asked Questions," National Council on Severe Autism, accessed August 29, 2019, https://www.ncsautism.org/faqs.

3 "Autism Facts and Figures," Autism Speaks, accessed September 4, 2019, https://www.autismspeaks.org/autism-facts-and-figures; Micah Mazurek, Stephen Kanne, and Ericka Wodka, "Physical Aggression in Children and Adolescents with Autism Spectrum Disorders," *Research in Autism Spectrum Disorders* 7, no. 3 (March 2013): 455.

4 Christa Holmans, "A Quick Note about 'Autism Martyr Parents,'" *Neurodivergent Rebel* (blog), March 5, 2018, https://neurodivergentrebel.com/2018/03/05/autism-martyr-parents/.

5 Michelle Diament, "Autism Moms Have Stress Similar to Combat Soldiers," *Disability Scoop*, November 10, 2009, https://www.disabilityscoop.com/2009/11/10/autism-moms-stress/6121/.

6 Lisa Freitag, *Extreme Caregiving: The Moral Work of Raising Children with Special Needs* (Oxford: Oxford University Press, 2018), 10.

7 Freitag, 35, 62.

8 Arthur Kleinman, *The Soul of Care: The Moral Education of a Husband and Doctor* (New York: Viking, 2019), 193.

9 Freitag, *Extreme Caregiving*, 1.

10 Kleinman, *Soul of Care*, 4.

11 Kleinman.

12 Joan Tronto, *Caring Democracy: Markets, Equality, and Justice* (New York: New York University Press, 2013), ix, 62.

1. We Walk

1 Victor Fleming, dir., *The Wizard of Oz* (Beverly Hills, CA: Metro-Goldwyn-Mayer, 1939), DVD.

2 "Books," *Elmo's World: Dancing, Music, Books*, directed by Ted May (1999; Burbank, CA: Warner Brothers Studio, 2010), DVD.

2. Physical Guidance

1 John Hardwig, "Epistemic Dependence," *Journal of Philosophy* 82, no. 7 (July 1985): 336.

2 Louis P. Hagopian, Samantha L. Hardesty, and Meagan Gregory, "Scientific Support for Applied Behavior Analysis from the Neurobehavioral Unit," accessed December 30, 2019, https://www.kennedykrieger.org/patient-care/centers-and-programs/neurobehavioral-unit-nbu/applied-behavior-analysis.

3 Michelle Dawson, "The Misbehaviour of Behaviourists: Ethical Challenges to the Autism-ABA Industry," *The Autism Crisis: Science and Ethics in the Era of Autism Advocacy* (blog), January 18, 2004, http://www.sentex.net/~nexus23/naa_aba.html.

4 Birdmad Girl, "I Abused Children for a Living," *Diary of a Birdmad Girl* (blog), April 3, 2017, https://madasbirdsblog.wordpress.com/2017/04/03/i-abused-children-for-a-living/.

5 Peter Gerhardt, "Adaptive Behavior and ASD: Life, Safety, Independence, and Community Competence" (presentation, International Conference for Autism, Antalya, Turkey, November 14–16, 2014), http://www.inca2014.com/sunular/ingilizce/Peter%20Gerhardt%20.pdf.

6 Elizabeth Devita-Raeburn, "The Controversy over Autism's Most Common Therapy," Spectrum, August 10, 2016, https://www.spectrumnews.org/features/deep-dive/controversy-autisms-common-therapy/.

7 Alison Singer, email message to author, October 5, 2017.

3. Answers and Questions

1 Amy S. F. Lutz, "Dear Stranger: Your Son's Autistic, Just Like Mine," *Babble*, September 13, 2007, https://www.babble.com/toddler/talking-to-parents-of-autistic-children-signs-of-autism-in-toddlers/.

2 Quoted in Maureen Dowd, "20 Years after the Murder of Kitty Genovese, the Question Remains: Why?," *New York Times*, March 12, 1984, https://www.nytimes.com/1984/03/12/nyregion/20-years-after-the-murder-of-kitty-genovese-the-question-remains-why.html.

3 Eugene Volokh, "Duty to Rescue/Report Statutes, " *The Volokh Conspiracy* (blog), November 3, 2009, http://volokh.com/2009/11/03/duty-to-rescuereport-statutes/.

4 Karen Alpert, "Dear Stranger Who Disciplined My Kiddo at the Playground Today," *Baby Sideburns* (blog), May 24, 2016, http://babysideburns.com/2016/05/playground-dicipline/.

5 *Beauty and the Beast*, directed by Gary Trousdale and Kirk Wise (1991; Burbank, CA: Walt Disney Studios), DVD.

6 Bryan Caplan, *The Myth of the Rational Voter: Why Democracies Choose Bad Policies* (Princeton, NJ: Princeton University Press, 2007), 116, 132.

7 Caplan, *Myth of the Rational Voter*, 135.

8 Quoted in Caplan, *Myth of the Rational Voter*, 136.

4. The Next Time

1 Amanda Van Allen, "Crying Child with Autism Kicked Out of Restaurant," 69 News, October 12, 2016, http://www.wfmz.com/news/southeastern-pa/crying-child-with-autism-kicked-out-of-restaurant_20161028031651547/133772765; Khaleda Rahman, "Mother of Autistic Boy Says She Was Humiliated after They Were Kicked Out of Pizza Restaurant Because He Was Being 'Too Loud,'" *Daily Mail*, October 9, 2016, http://www.dailymail.co.uk/news/article-3829500/Mother-autistic-boy-says-kicked-pizza-restaurant.html.

2 Sydney Lupkin and Emily Shapiro, "Mom of Girl with Autism Who Was Kicked off Plane Speaks Out," ABC News, May 11, 2015, http://abcnews.go.com/Health/mom-autistic-girl-kicked-off-plane-speaks/story?id=30965376; Heather Love, "Autistic Boy Thrown Out of Public Gardens for His Disability," YouTube, April 5, 2017, https://www.youtube.com/watch?v=Hsria6IFWXM; Siemny Kim, "Issaquah Mom Says Child with Autism Kicked Out of Movie Theater," Kiro 7, June 24, 2016, http://www.kiro7.com/news/local/mom-says-autistic-child-was-kicked-out-of-movie-theater/361901458.

3 Love, "Autistic Boy Thrown Out."

4 Susan Wendell, *The Rejected Body: Feminist Philosophical Reflections on Disability* (New York: Routledge, 1996), 60.

5 Edward O. Wilson, *The Meaning of Human Existence* (New York: Liveright, 2014), 24, 30.

6 Meagan M. Patterson and Rebecca S. Bigler, "Preschool Children's Attention to Environmental Messages about Groups: Social Categorization and the Origins of Intergroup Bias," *Child Development* 77 (2006): 847.

7 Henri Tajfel, "Experiments in Intergroup Discrimination," *Scientific American* 223, no. 5 (November 1970), 99, 101.

8 Philip Zimbardo, *The Lucifer Effect: Understanding How Good People Turn Evil* (New York: Random House, 2007).

9 Ellis M. Craig, "At the Dawn of Civilization: Intellectual Disability in Prehistory and Ancient Times (9000 to 500 CE)," in *The Story of Intellectual Disability: An Evolution of Meaning, Understanding, and Public Perception*, ed. Michael L. Wehmeyer (Baltimore: Paul H. Brookes, 2013), 26.

10 John Locke, *Essay Concerning Human Understanding* (London: Dent, 1961), 280.

11 Peter Singer, "All Animals Are Equal," in *Animal Rights and Human Obligations*, ed. Tom Regan and Peter Singer (Upper Saddle River, NJ: Prentice-Hall, 1989), 161.

12 Jeff McMahon, *The Ethics of Killing: Problems at the Margins of Life* (Oxford: Oxford University Press, 2002), 206.

13 Nora J. Baladerian, Thomas F. Coleman, and Jim Stream, *A Report on the 2012 National Survey on Abuse of People with Disabilities* (Spectrum Institute Disability and Abuse Project, 2013), 3, https://www.disabilityandabuse.org/survey/survey-report.pdf; Denise Valenti-Hein and Linda Schwartz, *The Sexual Abuse Interview for Those with Developmental Disabilities* (Santa Barbara, CA: James Stanfield, 1995), qtd. in Wisconsin Coalition Against Sexual Assault, *Sexual Assault and People with Developmental Disabilities: A Guide for Family Friends, and Caregivers* (brochure), 1997, www.ncdsv.org/images/SexAssaultandPeoplewith-Disabilities.pdf.

14 Michael J. Berens and Patricia Callahan, "Suffering in Secret: Illinois Hides Abuse and Neglect of Adults with Disabilities," *Chicago Tribune*, November 21, 2016, http://www.chicagotribune.com/news/watchdog/grouphomes/ct-group-home-investigations-cila-met-20161117-htmlstory.html.

15 Carolyn Gusoff, "Hamptons Group Home Workers Allegedly Ran 'Developmentally Disabled Fight Club,'" CBS New York, February 6, 2014, http://newyork.cbslocal.com/2014/02/06/long-island-group-home-workers-allegedly-forced-developmentally-disabled-people-to-fight/.

16 Zimbardo, *Lucifer Effect*, 307.

17 Shannon Des Roches Rosa, "*Rolling Stone*: Your Dehumanization of Autistic People Is the Problem," *Squidalicious* (blog), July 27, 2016, http://www.squidalicious.com/2016/07/rolling-stone-your-dehumanization-of.html; Emily Willingham, "*Rolling Stone* Offers Its Entry Into Parents-First Disability Genre," *Forbes*, July 27, 2016, https://www.forbes.com/sites/emilywillingham/2016/07/27/rolling-stone-offers-entry-into-parents-first-disability-genre/#3d699ec15bdf.

18 Paul Solotaroff, "Luke's Best Chance: One Man's Fight for His Autistic Son," *Rolling Stone*, July 27, 2016, https://www.rollingstone.com/culture/culture-features/lukes-best-chance-one-mans-fight-for-his-autistic-son-93049/.

19 Wendell, *Rejected Body*, 18.

20 Lisa Genova, *Still Alice* (New York: Pocket Books, 2007), 121.

21 John Wyatt, "What Is a Person?" *Nucleus*, Spring 2004: 10–15.

22 Eva Feder Kittay, "At the Margins of Moral Personhood," *Ethics* 116, no. 1 (October 2005): 122.

23 Eva Feder Kittay, "When Caring Is Just and Justice Is Caring: Justice and Mental Retardation," *Public Culture* 13, no. 3 (2001): 568.

24 Michael Bérubé, "Equality, Freedom, and/or Justice for All: A Response to Martha Nussbaum," in *Cognitive Disability and Its Challenge to Moral*

Philosophy, ed. Eva Feder Kittay and Licia Carlson (Chichester, UK: Wiley-Blackwell, 2010), 100.

25 Allison C. Carey, *On the Margins of Citizenship: Intellectual Disability and Civil Rights in Twentieth-Century America* (Philadelphia: Temple University Press, 2009), 227.

26 McMahan, *Ethics of Killing*, 147.

27 McMahan, *Ethics of Killing*, 222.

28 Kittay, "Margins," 122.

29 United Nations, "Universal Declaration of Human Rights," 2015, 1, https://www.un.org/en/udhrbook/pdf/udhr_booklet_en_web.pdf.

30 Steven Pinker, *The Blank Slate: The Modern Denial of Human Nature* (New York: Penguin Books, 2002), 320.

31 Peter Singer, *The Expanding Circle: Ethics, Evolution, and Moral Progress* (Princeton, NJ: Princeton University Press, 1981), 120.

32 Lauren Casper, "3 Responses for People Who Think My Son with Autism Shouldn't Go Out," The Mighty, June 17, 2015, https://themighty.com/2015/06/why-it-is-good-for-my-son-with-autism-to-go-out/.

33 A. Stout, "5 Reasons Why Your Child with Autism Needs to Be Out in Public," The Autism Site, accessed February 10, 2017, http://blog.theautismsite.com/seen-in-public/.

34 Philip G. Zimbardo and Michael R. Leippe, *The Psychology of Attitude Change and Social Influence* (New York: McGraw-Hill, 1991), 81.

35 K. Querry, "Heartwarming Promposal: Cheerleader Asks Boy with Autism to Prom," Oklahoma's News 4, February 23, 2016, http://kfor.com/2016/02/23/heartwarming-promposal-cheerleader-asks-boy-with-autism-to-prom/; David Williams, "Undefeated Wrestler Lets Opponent with Down Syndrome Win," CNN, January 28, 2016, http://www.cnn.com/2016/01/28/us/undefeated-wrestler-down-syndrome-irpt/index.html.

36 Kit Mead, "How the Media and Society Objectify Disabled People," *Paginated Thoughts* (blog), September 5, 2016, https://kpagination.wordpress.com/2016/09/05/how-media-and-society-objectify-disabled-people/.

37 "College Student Mows Hundreds of Lawns for Free while Teaching Values to Youth," Newsner, May 6, 2016, https://en.newsner.com/news/college-student-mows-hundreds-of-lawns-for-free-while-teaching-values-to-youth/; "Black Man Brings Starbucks to Police Guarding NYC Bombing Scene," The Grio, September 19, 2016, http://thegrio.com/2016/09/19/black-man-brings-starbucks-to-police-after-nyc-bombing/; Alexandra Zaslow, "Walmart Employee Gives Shoes off His Feet to Barefoot Homeless Man," *Today*, August 3, 2016, https://www.today.com/money/walmart-employee-gives-shoes-his-feet-barefoot-homeless-man-t101446.

38 Mary Bowerman, "Democrats Raise $13K to Reopen Firebombed GOP Headquarters," *USA Today*, October 17, 2016, https://www.usatoday.com/story/news/politics/onpolitics/2016/10/17/democrats-raise-13k-reopen-firebombed-gop-headquarters/92266000/.

39 David M. Perry, "How 'Inspiration Porn' Reporting Objectifies People with Disabilities," Medium, February 25, 2016, https://medium.com/the-establishment/how-inspiration-porn-reporting-objectifies-people-with-disabilities-db30023e3d2b.

40 Zimbardo, *Lucifer Effect*, 449.

41 Zimbardo and Leippe, *Psychology of Attitude Change*, 108.

42 Zimbardo and Leippe, *Psychology of Attitude Change*, 109.

43 Allen Buchanan, *Beyond Humanity* (Oxford: Oxford University Press, 2011), 231.

5. Just Say Yes

1 *The Simpsons*, season 7, episode 133, "Lisa the Vegetarian," directed by David S. Cohen, written by Mark Kirkland, aired October 15, 1995.

2 Jennifer Abbanat, in discussion with the author, August 11, 2017. All subsequent references are to this conversation.

3 U.S. Department of Health and Human Services, *Facing Addiction in America: The Surgeon General's Report on Alcohol, Drugs, and Health*, November 2016, https://www.ncbi.nlm.nih.gov/books/NBK424847/.

4 Rick Doblin, in discussion with the author, November 4, 2014. All subsequent references are to this conversation.

5 Casarett, David, *Stoned: A Doctor's Case for Medical Marijuana* (New York: Current, 2015), 254.

6 https://www.ncbi.nlm.nih.gov/pubmed.

7 Madeline H. Meier et al., "Persistent Cannabis Users Show Neuropsychological Decline from Childhood to Midlife," *Proceedings of the National Academy of Sciences* 109, no. 4 (October 2, 2012), http://www.pnas.org/content/109/40/E2657/tab-article-info.

8 Christopher Ingraham, "Scientists Have Found That Smoking Weed Does Not Make You Stupid after All," *Washington Post*, January 18, 2016, https://www.washingtonpost.com/news/wonk/wp/2016/01/18/scientists-have-found-that-smoking-weed-does-not-make-you-stupid-after-all/.

9 Lester Grinspoon, in discussion with the author, July 23, 2014.

10 John Williams, in discussion with the author, October 9, 2014.

11 Kevin Gray, in discussion with the author, May 7, 2015.

12 Casarett, *Stoned*, 140.

13 Williams, in discussion with the author, October 9, 2014.

14 Csaba Földy, Robert C. Malenka, and Thomas C. Südhof, "Autism-Associated Neuroligin-3 Mutations Commonly Disrupt Tonic Endocannabinoid Signaling," *Neuron* 78 (May 8, 2013): 498.

15 Marilyn Elias, "New Antipsychotic Drugs Carry Risks for Children," *USA Today*, May 2, 2006; Gardiner Harris, Benedict Carey, and Janet Roberts,

"Psychiatrists, Children, and Drug Industry's Role," *New York Times*, May 10, 2007, https://www.nytimes.com/2007/05/10/health/10psyche.html.

16 Christoph U. Correll et al., "Cardiometabolic Risk of Second-Generation Antipsychotic Medications during First-Time Use in Children and Adolescents," *Journal of the American Medical Association* 302, no. 16 (2009): 1765.

17 Gray, in discussion with the author, May 7, 2015.

18 Jonathan Moreno, in discussion with the author, September 30, 2014.

19 Grinspoon, in discussion with the author, July 23, 2014.

20 Karen Echols, in discussion with the author, August 2, 2014.

21 Tara, in discussion with the author, August 13, 2014.

22 Tara, Facebook message to the author, July 31, 2017.

23 Casarett, *Stoned*, 238, 249. THC and CBD are the two most abundant cannabinoids in marijuana.

24 Casarett, *Stoned*, 241.

25 Grinspoon, in discussion with the author, July 23, 2014.

26 Grinspoon, in discussion with the author, July 23, 2014.

27 Stephanie Lay, in discussion with the author, July 24, 2014.

28 Gray, in discussion with the author, May 7, 2015.

29 Autism Speaks, "Consensus Conference: Identifying Next Steps in Research on Cannabis and Autism," New York City, November 29–30, 2018. This conference included thirty-six physicians, researchers, parents, providers, and members of the Autism Speaks staff and featured presentations and breakout groups. A PDF copy of the conference proposal is available at https://www.autismspeaks.org/sites/default/files/Cannabis Research Consensus Conference (3).pdf.

6. All Possible Spaces

1 Amanda Moseley, email to author, November 4, 2018.

2 Robert L. Selman, *The Growth of Interpersonal Understanding: Developmental and Clinical Analyses* (New York: Academic Press, 1980), 37.

3 Amy S. F. Lutz, "Friends for Hire? For Those with Severe I/DD, Relationships with Direct Care Staff Are Primary," *Psychology Today*, October 14, 2018, https://www.psychologytoday.com/us/blog/inspectrum/201810/friends-hire.

4 Kaitlin Coryat Fernandez, email to author, November 8, 2018. In the skit she describes, Kermit goes to a shop to pick up a "Kermit the Frog" T-shirt he has ordered. The clerk pulls out a series of shirts with *frog* misspelled. Each time, with increasing agitation, Kermit accuses the clerk of spelling his name wrong, and each time a different Muppet shows up to claim the shirt. Finally, after Kermit screams, "My name is Kermit the Frog and I want my Kermit the Frog T-shirt," the clerk informs him that his order won't be ready until Tuesday. *The Best of Kermit*, directed by John Chiappardi (New York, NY: Sony Wonder, 1998), VHS.

5 Aristotle, Ethics (Pantianos Classics, 1908), 119.

6 Aristotle, *Ethics*, 121.

7 Michel de Montaigne, "Of Friendship," in Works of Michel de Montaigne: Comprising His Essays, Journey into Italy, and Letters, ed. William Hazlitt (Boston, MA: Houghton, Osgood and Company, 1879), 276.

8 Mark Vernon, *The Meaning of Friendship* (Basingstoke: Palgrave Macmillan, 2010), 224.

9 Aristotle, *Ethics*, 121.

10 Alexander Nehamas, *On Friendship* (New York: Basic Books, 2016), 112.

11 Nehamas, *On Friendship*, 210.

12 Ben Kaliner, email to author, November 26, 2018.

13 Autistic Self-Advocacy Network, Self Advocates Becoming Empowered, and the National Youth Leadership Network, "Keeping the Promise: Self Advocates Defining the Meaning of Community Living," accessed December 15, 2018, https://autisticadvocacy.org/wp-content/uploads/2012/02/KeepingthePromise SelfAdvocatesDefiningtheMeaningofCommunity.pdf.

14 Lucy Hurst-Brown, "People with Learning Disabilities Need Friends, Not Just Paid Carers," *The Guardian*, October 23, 2014, https://www.the-guardian.com/social-care-network/2014/oct/23/people-learning-disabilities-community.

15 Donna Thomson, "Can Paid Caregivers Also Be Friends?" Dugan Disability Law, accessed December 18, 2018, https://getdisabilitysocialsecurity.com/dugandisabilitylaw/can-paid-caregivers-also-friends/.

16 Liz Spencer and Ray Pahl, *Rethinking Friendship: Hidden Solidarities Today* (Princeton, NJ: Princeton University Press, 2006), 84.

17 Spencer and Pahl, 192.

18 Ashley Bockman, Facebook message to author, November 14, 2018.

19 Tom Wolf, "Executive Order: 2016-03: Establishing 'Employment First' Policy and Increasing Competitive Integrated Employment for Pennsylvanians with a Disability," March 10, 2016, https://www.governor.pa.gov/newsroom/executive-order-2016-03-establishing-employment-first-policy-increasing-competitive-integrated-employment-pennsylvanians-disability/.

20 National Council on Disability, "NCD Policy Areas," accessed December 2, 2018, https://ncd.gov/.

21 Judith Graham, "Severe Shortage of Direct Care Workers Triggering Crisis," Disability Scoop, May 9, 2017, https://www.disabilityscoop.com/2017/05/09/severe-shortage-care-crisis/23679/.

22 Baladerian, Coleman, and Stream, *A Report on the 2012 National Survey on Abuse of People with Disabilities*, 3.

23 Jessica Zawacki, email to author, October 31, 2019.

24 *The Best of Ernie and Bert*, directed by Jon Stone (1988; Los Angeles, CA: Random House Home Video, 2003), DVD.

25 Spencer and Pahl, *Rethinking Friendship*, 58.

26 Michel Foucault, "Friendship as a Way of Life," *Le gai pied*, April 1981, translation by John Johnston, posted on Caring Labor: An Archive, November 18, 2010, https://caringlabor.wordpress.com/2010/11/18/michel-foucault-friendship-as-a-way-of-life/.

27 Nick Taugner, email to author, November 6, 2018.

7. Praesidalism

1 "Portrayal of People with Disabilities," Association of University Centers on Disabilities, accessed 10/1/17, http://www.aucd.org/template/page.cfm?id=605.

2 Lydia Brown, "The Significance of Semantics: Person-First Language: Why It Matters," *Autistic Hoya* (blog), August 4, 2011, http://www.autistichoya.com/2011/08/significance-of-semantics-person-first.html.

3 Stuart Duncan, "The Last Word on 'Person First Language,'" *Autism from a Father's Point of View* (blog), July 12, 2011, http://www.stuartduncan.name/autism/the-last-word-on-person-first-language/.

4 Jim Endersby, *Imperial Nature: Joseph Hooker and the Practices of Victorian Science* (Chicago: University of Chicago Press, 2008), 27.

5 Bryan King, in discussion with the author, May 2, 2013.

6 Catherine Lord et al., "A Multisite Study of the Clinical Diagnoses of Different Autism Spectrum Disorders," *Archives of General Psychiatry* 69, no. 3 (March 2012): 306.

7 Qtd. in "Aspie Bigotry at Autism Speaks Blog," *Autism Jabberwocky* (blog), September 26, 2010, http://autismjabberwocky.blogspot.com/2010/09/aspie-bigotry-at-autism-speaks-blog.html.

8 Tom Hibben, in discussion with the author, May 2, 2013.

9 Francesca Happé, "Why Fold Asperger Syndrome into Autism Spectrum Disorder in the DSM-5," Spectrum, March 29, 2011, https://www.spectrumnews.org/opinion/viewpoint/why-fold-asperger-syndrome-into-autism-spectrum-disorder-in-the-dsm-5/.

10 Judith Ursitti, in conversation with the author, May 2, 2013.

11 Simon Baron-Cohen, "The Short Life of a Diagnosis," *New York Times*, November 9, 2009, https://www.nytimes.com/2009/11/10/opinion/10baron-cohen.html.

12 D. M. Kite, J. Gullifer, and G. A. Tyson, "Views on the Diagnostic Labels of Autism and Asperger's Disorder and the Proposed Changes in the DSM," *Journal of Autism and Developmental Disorders* 43, no. 7 (July 2013): 1692–700.

13 Luke Y. Tsai, "Asperger's Disorder Will Be Back," *Journal of Autism and Developmental Disorders* 43 (2013): 2916.

14 Qtd. in "World's Largest Autism Genome Database Shines New Light on Many 'Autisms,'" Autism Speaks, March 6, 2017, https://www.autismspeaks.org/science-news/worlds-largest-autism-genome-database-shines-new-light-many-autisms.

15 Qtd. in "Probing the Mysterious Perceptual World of Autism," Caltech, October 22, 2015, http://www.caltech.edu/news/probing-mysterious-perceptual-world-autism-48543.

16 Greg Boustead, "IMFAR 2013: Autism or 'Autisms'?" Spectrum, May 6, 2013, https://spectrumnews.org/news/imfar-2013-autism-or-autisms/.

17 Marie Myung-Ok Lee, "Jerry Seinfeld's Not Helping: Celebrity Autism Claims Distract from Reality and Research," Salon, November 10, 2014, https://www.salon.com/2014/11/10/jerry_seinfelds_not_helping_celebrities_with_autism_distract_from_reality_and_research/.

18 Lydia Brown, "So High-Functioning (Sarcasm)," *Autistic Hoya* (blog), September 26, 2012, https://www.autistichoya.com/2012/09/so-high-functioning-sarcasm.html.

19 Cynthia Kim, "Decoding the High Functioning Label," *Musings of an Aspie* (blog), June 26, 2013, https://musingsofanaspie.com/2013/06/26/decoding-the-high-functioning-label/.

20 Qtd. in Andrew Solomon, "The Autism Rights Movement," *New York*, May 25, 2008, http://nymag.com/news/features/47225/.

21 Feda Almaliti, "Inclusion Sucks. Or, Why My Son with Severe Autism Has Nowhere to Swim This Summer," Autism Society San Francisco Bay Area, July 25, 2017, http://www.sfautismsociety.org/blog/inclusion-sucks-or-why-my-son-with-severe-autism-has-nowhere-to-swim-this-summer.

22 Julia Bascom, "Dear 'Autism Parents,'" *Just Stimming* (blog), August 23, 2011, https://juststimming.wordpress.com/2011/08/23/dear-autism-parents/.

23 Sara Luterman, "Autistic Advocates Clash with Autism Parents at Government Committee Meeting," NOS Magazine, October 27, 2017, http://nosmag.org/parents-and-autistic-adults-clash-at-autism-committee-meeting-iacc-interagency-autism-coordinating-committee/.

24 Quoted in Luterman, "Autistic Advocates Clash."

25 Amy S.F. Lutz, "Who Decides Where Autistic Adults Live?" *The Atlantic*, May 26, 2015, https://www.theatlantic.com/health/archive/2015/05/who-decides-where-autistic-adults-live/393455/.

26 D.A. Sisti, A.G. Segal, and E.J. Emanuel, "Improving Long-Term Psychiatric Care: Bring Back the Asylum," *Journal of the American Medical Association* 313, no. 3 (2015): 244.

27 Dominic Sisti, in discussion with the author, February 5, 2014.

28 Harlan Hahn, "Accommodations and the ADA: Unreasonable Bias or Biased Reasoning?," *Berkeley Journal of Employment and Labor Law* 166 (2000): 181.

29 Philip M. Ferguson, "The Social Construction of Mental Retardation," *Social Policy* 18, no. 1 (July 1987): 56.

30 "Toward Autonomy and Self-Determination—World Autism Awareness Day 2017," UN Web TV, March 31, 2017, http://webtv.un.org/search/toward-autonomy-and-self-determination-world-autism-awareness-day-2017/5380816054001.

31 Paul S. Appelbaum, "There Are All Kinds of Rights," *Hastings Center Report* 46, no. 2 (March/April 2016): inside back cover.

32 "Carol Gilligan Interview," Ethics of Care, June 21, 2011, https://ethicsofcare.org/carol-gilligan/.

33 Eva Feder Kittay, *Love's Labor: Essays on Women, Equality, and Dependency* (New York: Routledge, 1999), 5.

34 Kittay, *Love's Labor*, 66.

35 Kittay, *Love's Labor*, 107.

36 Sandra Laugier, "The Ethics of Care as a Politics of the Ordinary," *New Literary History* 46, no. 2 (Spring 2015): 221, 227.

8. The Child Who Does Not Know How to Ask

1 The Jewish Federations of North America, *The Passover Haggadah: A Guide to the Seder*, accessed October 28, 2016, http://jewishfederation.org/images/uploads/holiday_images/39497.pdf.

2 *Tanakh: The Holy Scriptures* (Philadelphia: The Jewish Publication Society, 1988).

3 *The New Testament in Modern English*, trans. J. B. Phillips (New York: Macmillan, 1958).

4 Craig, "Dawn of Civilization," 21.

5 Stephen Bramer, "Suffering in the Pentateuch," in *Why, O God? Suffering and Disability in the Bible and Church*, ed. Larry J. Waters and Roy B. Zuck (Wheaton, IL: Crossway, 2011), 88; Stephanie O. Hubach, *Same Lake, Different Boat: Coming alongside People Touched by Disability* (Phillipsburg, NJ: P & R, 2006), 27.

6 Larry J. Waters, "Suffering in the Book of Job," in Waters and Zuck, *Why, O God?*, 120.

7 Joni Tada Eareckson, "Wheelchairs in Heaven?," in Waters and Zuck, *Why, O God?*, 324.

8 Kelly Langston, *Autism's Hidden Blessings: Discovering God's Promises for Autistic Children & Their Families* (Grand Rapids, MI: Kregel, 2009), 185.

9 Kathy Medina, *Finding God in Autism: A 40 Day Devotional for Parents of Autistic Spectrum Children* (Mustang, OK: Tate, 2006), 49.

10 Christopher De Vinck, *The Power of the Powerless: A Brother's Legacy of Love* (New York: Crossroad, 1988), 105.

11 Qtd. in De Vinck, *Power of the Powerless*, xvi.

12 Harold S. Kushner, *When Bad Things Happen to Good People* (New York: Anchor Books, 1981), 29, 35.

13 Langston, *Autism's Hidden Blessings*, 26.

14 Michael A. Justice, "Disabilities and the Church," in Waters and Zuck, *Why, O God?*, 56.

15 Douglas K. Blount, "Receiving Evil from God," in Waters and Zuck, *Why, O God?*, 219.

16 Langston, *Autism's Hidden Blessings*, 121.

17 Kushner, *When Bad Things Happen*, 147.

18 Andrew Griffin, "Elon Musk: The Chance We Are Not Living in a Computer Simulation is 'One in Billions,'" *Independent*, June 2, 2016, https://www.independent.co.uk/life-style/gadgets-and-tech/news/elon-musk-ai-artificial-intelligence-computer-simulation-gaming-virtual-reality-a7060941.html.

19 Émile Durkheim, *The Elementary Forms of Religious Life* (Oxford: Oxford University Press, 2001), xxiii.

20 Durkheim, 258.

21 Debbie, in discussion with the author, September 26, 2016.

22 Susan Senator, in discussion with the author, September 23, 2016.

23 Durkheim, 170.

9. Baseline

1 Our ECT journey is recounted in Amy S. F. Lutz, *Each Day I Like it Better: Autism, ECT, and the Treatment of Our Most Impaired Children* (Nashville: Vanderbilt University Press, 2014).

2 Robert Berezin, "No, There Is No Such Thing as ADHD," *Psychology Today*, March 17, 2015, https://www.psychologytoday.com/us/blog/the-theater-the-brain/201503/no-there-is-no-such-thing-adhd.

3 Hanif Kureishi, "The Art of Distraction," *New York Times*, February 18, 2012, https://www.nytimes.com/2012/02/19/opinion/sunday/the-art-of-distraction.html.

4 Marilyn Wedge, *Suffer the Children: The Case against Labeling and Medicating and an Effective Alternative* (New York: W. W. Norton, 2011), 5.

5 Claudia M. Gold, *The Silenced Child: From Labels, Medications, and Quick-Fix Solutions to Listening, Growth, and Lifelong Resilience* (Boston: Da Capo Press, 2016), xxv.

6 Gold, *Silenced Child*, 211.

7 Michael Schofield, *January First* (New York: Crown, 2012); Lutz, *Each Day I Like It Better*, chapter 8.

8 Gold, *Silenced Child*, 75.

9 Berezin, "No, There Is No Such Thing as ADHD."

10 Bruno Bettelheim, *The Empty Fortress* (New York: Simon and Schuster, 1972), 125.

11 Wedge, *Suffer the Children*, 2; Francis Fukuyama, *Our Posthuman Future* (New York: Picador, 2002), 49.

12 "International Consensus Statement on ADHD," *Clinical Child and Family Psychology Review* 5, no. 2 (June 2002): 91.

13 Russell A. Barkley, Edwin H. Cook, Jr., Adele Diamond, et al., "International Consensus Statement on ADHD," *Clinical Child and Family Psychology Review* 5, no. 2 (June 2002): 90.

14 Alan Schwarz, *ADHD Nation: Children, Doctors, Big Pharma, and the Making of an American Epidemic* (New York: Scribner, 2016), 1.

15 Gold, *Silenced Child*, 114; Peter Breggin, *Reclaiming Our Children: A Healing Plan for a Nation in Crisis* (Boston: DaCapo, 2000), 142.

16 Jason Padgett and Maureen Seaberg, *Struck by Genius: How a Brain Injury Made Me a Mathematical Marvel* (Boston: Houghton Mifflin, 2014), 6, 148.

17 *Regarding Henry*, directed by Mike Nichols (1991; Hollywood, CA: Paramount Pictures); Lisa Genova, *Still Alice* (New York, NY: Gallery Books, 2009).

18 Gilbert Ryle, *The Concept of Mind* (Chicago: University of Chicago Press, 2000), 15.

19 Michael S. Gazzaniga, *Who's in Charge? Free Will and the Science of the Brain* (New York: Ecco, 2011), 102.

20 Gazzaniga, *Who's in Charge?*, 87.

21 Gazzaniga, *Who's in Charge?*, 90.

22 Yuval Noah Harari, *Homo Deus: A Brief History of Tomorrow* (New York: Harper, 2017), 301.

23 Gazzaniga, *Who's in Charge?*, 63.

24 Harari, *Homo Deus*, 292.

25 Ilina Singh, "Not Robots: Children's Perspectives on Authenticity, Moral Agency and Stimulant Drug Treatments," *Journal of Medical Ethics* 39, no. 6 (August 28, 2012), http://jme.bmj.com/content/early/2012/08/27/medethics-2011-100224.

26 Peter Kramer, *Listening to Prozac* (New York: Penguin Books, 1993), 8, 147, 19.

27 Adrian Raine, *The Anatomy of Violence: The Biological Roots of Crime* (New York: Pantheon Books, 2013), 316.

28 G. E. Moore, *Principia Ethica* (Cambridge: Cambridge University Press, 1903), 44.

29 Fukuyama, *Our Posthuman Future*, 47.

30 Gazzaniga, *Who's in Charge?*, 75.

Bibliography

Almaliti, Feda. "Inclusion Sucks. Or, Why My Son with Severe Autism Has Nowhere to Swim This Summer." Autism Society San Francisco Bay Area, July 25, 2017. http://www.sfautismsociety.org/blog/inclusion-sucks-or-why-my-son-with-severe-autism-has-nowhere-to-swim-this-summer.

Alpert, Karen. "Dear Stranger Who Disciplined My Kiddo at the Playground Today." *Baby Sideburns* (blog), May 24, 2016. http://babysideburns.com/2016/05/playground-dicipline/.

Appelbaum, Paul S. "There Are All Kinds of Rights." *Hastings Center Report* 46, no. 2 (March/April 2016): inside back cover.

Aristotle, *Ethics*. Pantianos Classics, 1908.

"Aspie Bigotry at Autism Speaks Blog." *Autism Jabberwocky* (blog), September 26, 2010. http://autismjabberwocky.blogspot.com/2010/09/aspie-bigotry-at-autism-speaks-blog.html.

Association of University Centers on Disabilities. "Portrayal of People with Disabilities," accessed October 1, 2017. http://www.aucd.org/template/page.cfm?id=605.

Autism Speaks. "Autism Facts and Figures," accessed September 4, 2019. https://www.autismspeaks.org/autism-facts-and-figures.

———. "World's Largest Autism Genome Database Shines New Light on Many 'Autisms." March 6, 2017. https://www.autismspeaks.org/science-news/worlds-largest-autism-genome-database-shines-new-light-many-autisms.

Autistic Self-Advocacy Network, Self Advocates Becoming Empowered, and the National Youth Leadership Network. "Keeping the Promise: Self Advocates Defining the Meaning of Community Living," accessed December 15, 2018. https://autisticadvocacy.org/wp-content/uploads/2012/02/KeepingthePromise-SelfAdvocatesDefiningtheMeaningofCommunity.pdf.

Baladerian, Nora J., Thomas F. Coleman, and Jim Stream. *A Report on the 2012 National Survey on Abuse of People with Disabilities.* Spectrum Institute Disability and Abuse Project, 2013. https://disabilityandabuse.org/survey/survey-report.pdf.

Barkley, Russell A., Edwin H. Cook, Jr., Adele Diamond, et al. "International Consensus Statement on ADHD." *Clinical Child and Family Psychology Review* 5, no. 2 (June 2002): 89-111.

Baron-Cohen, Simon. "The Short Life of a Diagnosis." *New York Times*, November 9, 2009. https://www.nytimes.com/2009/11/10/opinion/10baron-cohen.html.

Bascom, Julia. "Dear 'Autism Parents.'" *Just Stimming* (blog), August 23, 2011. https://juststimming.wordpress.com/2011/08/23/dear-autism-parents/.

Berens, Michael J., and Patricia Callahan. "Suffering in Secret: Illinois Hides Abuse and Neglect of Adults with Disabilities." *Chicago Tribune*, November 21, 2016. http://www.chicagotribune.com/news/watchdog/grouphomes/ct-group-home-investigations-cila-met-20161117-htmlstory.html.

Berezin, Robert. "No, There Is No Such Thing as ADHD." *Psychology Today*, March 17, 2015. https://www.psychologytoday.com/us/blog/the-theater-the-brain/201503/no-there-is-no-such-thing-adhd.

Bérubé, Michael. "Equality, Freedom, and/or Justice for All: A Response to Martha Nussbaum." In *Cognitive Disability and Its Challenge to Moral Philosophy*, edited by Eva Feder Kittay and Licia Carlson, 97–109. Chichester: Wiley-Blackwell, 2010.

The Best of Kermit, directed by John Chiappardi (New York, NY: Sony Wonder, 1998), VHS.

Bettelheim, Bruno. *The Empty Fortress.* New York, NY: Simon and Schuster, 1972.

Birdmad Girl. "I Abused Children for a Living." *Diary of a Birdmad Girl* (blog), April 3, 2017. https://madasbirdsblog.wordpress.com/2017/04/03/i-abused-children-for-a-living/.

"Black Man Brings Starbucks to Police Guarding NYC Bombing Scene." The Grio, September 19, 2016. http://thegrio.com/2016/09/19/black-man-brings-starbucks-to-police-after-nyc-bombing/.

Blount, Douglas K. "Receiving Evil from God." In Waters and Zuck, *Why, O God?*, 217–29.

Boustead, Greg. "IMFAR 2013: Autism or 'Autisms'?" Spectrum, May 6, 2013. https://spectrumnews.org/news/imfar-2013-autism-or-autisms/.

Bowerman, Mary. "Democrats Raise $13K to Reopen Firebombed GOP Headquarters." *USA Today*, October 17, 2016. https://www.usatoday.com/

story/news/politics/onpolitics/2016/10/17/democrats-raise-13k-reopen-firebombed-gop-headquarters/92266000/.

Bramer, Stephen. "Suffering in the Pentateuch." In Waters and Zuck, *Why, O God?*, 87–97.

Breggin, Peter. *Reclaiming Our Children: A Healing Plan for a Nation in Crisis.* Boston: DaCapo, 2000.

Brown, Lydia. "The Significance of Semantics: Person-First Language: Why It Matters." *Autistic Hoya* (blog), August 4, 2011. http://www.autistichoya.com/2011/08/significance-of-semantics-person-first.html.

———. "So High-Functioning (Sarcasm)." *Autistic Hoya* (blog), September 26, 2012. https://www.autistichoya.com/2012/09/so-high-functioning-sarcasm.html.

Buchanan, Allen. *Beyond Humanity?* Oxford: Oxford University Press, 2011.

Caplan, Bryan. *The Myth of the Rational Voter: Why Democracies Choose Bad Policies.* Princeton, NJ: Princeton University Press, 2007.

Carey, Allison C. *On the Margins of Citizenship: Intellectual Disability and Civil Rights in Twentieth-Century America.* Philadelphia: Temple University Press, 2009.

"Carol Gilligan Interview." Ethics of Care, June 21, 2011. https://ethicsofcare.org/carol-gilligan/.

Casarett, David. *Stoned: A Doctor's Case for Medical Marijuana.* New York: Current, 2015.

Casper, Lauren. "3 Responses for People Who Think My Son with Autism Shouldn't Go Out." The Mighty, June 17, 2015. https://themighty.com/2015/06/why-it-is-good-for-my-son-with-autism-to-go-out/.

Cohen, David S., dir. *The Simpsons.* Season 7, episode 133, "Lisa the Vegetarian." Aired October 15, 1995 on Fox.

"College Student Mows Hundreds of Lawns for Free while Teaching Values to Youth." Newsner, May 6, 2016. https://en.newsner.com/news/college-student-mows-hundreds-of-lawns-for-free-while-teaching-values-to-youth/.

Correll, Christoph U., Peter Manu, Vladimir Olshanskiy, Barbara Napolitano, John M. Kane, and Anil K. Malhotra. "Cardiometabolic Risk of Second-Generation Antipsychotic Medications during First-Time Use in Children and Adolescents." *Journal of the American Medical Association* 302, no. 16 (2009): 1765–73.

Craig, Ellis M. "At the Dawn of Civilization: Intellectual Disability in Prehistory and Ancient Times (9000 to 500 CE)." In *The Story of Intellectual Disability: An Evolution of Meaning, Understanding, and Public Perception*, edited by Michael L. Wehmeyer, 19–46. Baltimore: Paul H. Brookes, 2013.

Dawson, Michelle. "The Misbehaviour of Behaviourists: Ethical Challenges to the Autism-ABA Industry." *The Autism Crisis: Science and Ethics in the Era of Autism Advocacy* (blog), January 18, 2004. http://www.sentex.net/~nexus23/naa_aba.html.

De Vinck, Christopher. *The Power of the Powerless: A Brother's Legacy of Love.* New York: Crossroad, 1988.

Devita-Raeburn, Elizabeth. "The Controversy over Autism's Most Common Therapy." Spectrum, August 10, 2016. https://www.spectrumnews.org/features/deep-dive/controversy-autisms-common-therapy/.

Diament, Michelle. "Autism Moms Have Stress Similar to Combat Soldiers." Disability Scoop, November 10, 2009. https://www.disabilityscoop.com/2009/11/10/autism-moms-stress/6121/.

Dowd, Maureen. "20 Years after the Murder of Kitty Genovese, the Question Remains: Why?" *New York Times*, March 12, 1984. https://www.nytimes.com/1984/03/12/nyregion/20-years-after-the-murder-of-kitty-genovese-the-question-remains-why.html.

Duncan, Stuart. "The Last Word on 'Person First Language.'" *Autism from a Father's Point of View* (blog), July 12, 2011. http://www.stuartduncan.name/autism/the-last-word-on-person-first-language/.

Durkheim, Émile. *The Elementary Forms of Religious Life.* Oxford: Oxford University Press, 2001.

Eareckson Tada, Joni. "Wheelchairs in Heaven?" In Waters and Zuck, *Why, O God?*, 315–24.

Elias, Marilyn. "New Antipsychotic Drugs Carry Risks for Children." *USA Today*, May 2, 2006.

Endersby, Jim. *Imperial Nature: Joseph Hooker and the Practices of Victorian Science.* Chicago: University of Chicago Press, 2008.

Ferguson, Philip M. "The Social Construction of Mental Retardation." *Social Policy* 18, no. 1 (July 1987): 51–56.

Földy, Csaba, Robert C. Malenka, and Thomas C. Südhof. "Autism-Associated Neuroligin-3 Mutations Commonly Disrupt Tonic Endocannabinoid Signaling." *Neuron* 78 (May 8, 2013): 498–509.

Foucault, Michel. "Friendship as a Way of Life." *Le gai pied*, April 1981. Translation by John Johnston posted on Caring Labor: An Archive, November 18, 2010. https://caringlabor.wordpress.com/2010/11/18/michel-foucault-friendship-as-a-way-of-life/.

Freitag, Lisa. *Extreme Caregiving: The Moral Work of Raising Children with Special Needs.* Oxford: Oxford University Press, 2018.

Fukuyama, Francis. *Our Posthuman Future.* New York: Picador, 2002.

Gazzaniga, Michael S. *Who's in Charge? Free Will and the Science of the Brain.* New York: Ecco, 2011.

Genova, Lisa. *Still Alice.* New York: Gallery Books, 2009.

Gerhardt, Peter. "Adaptive Behavior and ASD: Life, Safety, Independence, and Community Competence." Presentation, International Conference for Autism, Antalya, Turkey, November 14–16, 2014. http://www.inca2014.com/sunular/ingilizce/Peter%20Gerhardt%20.pdf.

Gold, Claudia M. *The Silenced Child: From Labels, Medications, and Quick-Fix Solutions to Listening, Growth, and Lifelong Resilience.* Boston: Da Capo Press, 2016.

Graham, Judith. "Severe Shortage of Direct Care Workers Triggering Crisis." Disability Scoop, May 9, 2017. https://www.disabilityscoop.com/2017/05/09/severe-shortage-care-crisis/23679/.

Griffin, Andrew. "Elon Musk: The Chance We Are Not Living in a Computer Simulation is 'One in Billions.'" Independent, June 2, 2016. https://www.independent.co.uk/life-style/gadgets-and-tech/news/elon-musk-ai-artificial-intelligence-computer-simulation-gaming-virtual-reality-a7060941.html.

Gusoff, Carolyn. "Hamptons Group Home Workers Allegedly Ran 'Developmentally Disabled Fight Club.'" CBS New York, February 6, 2014. http://newyork.cbslocal.com/2014/02/06/long-island-group-home-workers-allegedly-forced-developmentally-disabled-people-to-fight/.

Hagopian, Louis P., Samantha L. Hardesty, and Meagan Gregory. "Scientific Support for Applied Behavior Analysis from the Neurobehavioral Unit." Accessed December 30, 2019. https://www.kennedykrieger.org/patient-care/centers-and-programs/neurobehavioral-unit-nbu/applied-behavior-analysis.

Hahn, Harlan. "Accommodations and the ADA: Unreasonable Bias or Biased Reasoning?" *Berkeley Journal of Employment and Labor Law* 166 (2000): 166–92.

Happé, Francesca. "Why Fold Asperger Syndrome Into Autism Spectrum Disorder in the DSM-5." Spectrum, March 29, 2011. https://www.spectrumnews.org/opinion/viewpoint/why-fold-asperger-syndrome-into-autism-spectrum-disorder-in-the-dsm-5/.

Harari, Yuval Noah. *Homo Deus: A Brief History of Tomorrow.* New York: Harper, 2017.

Hardwig, John. "Epistemic Dependence." *Journal of Philosophy* 82, no. 7 (July 1985): 335–49.

Harris, Gardiner, Benedict Carey, and Janet Roberts. "Psychiatrists, Children, and Drug Industry's Role." *New York Times*, May 10, 2007. https://www.nytimes.com/2007/05/10/health/10psyche.html.

Holmans, Christa. "A Quick Note about 'Autism Martyr Parents.'" *Neurodivergent Rebel* (blog), March 5, 2018. https://neurodivergentrebel.com/2018/03/05/autism-martyr-parents/.

Hubach, Stephanie O. *Same Lake, Different Boat: Coming alongside People Touched by Disability*. Phillipsburg, NJ: P & R, 2006.

Hurst-Brown, Lucy. "People with Learning Disabilities Need Friends, Not Just Paid Carers." *The Guardian*, October 23, 2014. https://www.theguardian.com/social-care-network/2014/oct/23/people-learning-disabilities-community.

Ingraham, Christopher. "Scientists Have Found That Smoking Weed Does Not Make You Stupid after All." *Washington Post*, January 18, 2016. https://www.washingtonpost.com/news/wonk/wp/2016/01/18/scientists-have-found-that-smoking-weed-does-not-make-you-stupid-after-all/.

"International Consensus Statement on ADHD." *Clinical Child and Family Psychology Review* 5, no. 2 (June 2002): 89–111.

Jewish Federations of North America. *The Passover Haggadah: A Guide to the Seder*, accessed October 28, 2016. http://jewishfederation.org/images/uploads/holiday_images/39497.pdf.

Justice, Michael A. "Disabilities and the Church." In Waters and Zuck, *Why, O God?*, 55–67.

Kaufman, Joanne. "Ransom-Note Ads about Children's Health Are Canceled." *New York Times*, December 20, 2007. https://www.nytimes.com/2007/12/20/business/media/20child.html.

Kim, Cynthia. "Decoding the High Functioning Label." *Musings of an Aspie* (blog), June 26, 2013. https://musingsofanaspie.com/2013/06/26/decoding-the-high-functioning-label/.

Kim, Siemny. "Issaquah Mom Says Child with Autism Kicked Out of Movie Theater." Kiro 7, June 24, 2016. http://www.kiro7.com/news/local/mom-says-autistic-child-was-kicked-out-of-movie-theater/361901458.

Kite, D. M., J. Gullifer, and G. A. Tyson. "Views on the Diagnostic Labels of Autism and Asperger's Disorder and the Proposed Changes in the DSM." *Journal of Autism and Developmental Disorders* 43, no. 7 (July 2013): 1692–700.

Kittay, Eva Feder. "At the Margins of Moral Personhood." *Ethics* 116, no. 1 (October 2005): 100–31.

———. *Love's Labor: Essays on Women, Equality, and Dependency*. New York: Routledge, 1999.

———. "When Caring Is Just and Justice Is Caring: Justice and Mental Retardation." *Public Culture* 13, no. 3 (2001): 557–79.

Kleinman, Arthur. *The Soul of Care: The Moral Education of a Husband and Doctor*. New York: Viking, 2019.

Kramer, Peter. *Listening to Prozac*. New York: Penguin Books, 1993.

Kureishi, Hanif. "The Art of Distraction." *New York Times*, February 18, 2012. https://www.nytimes.com/2012/02/19/opinion/sunday/the-art-of-distraction.html.

Kushner, Harold S. *When Bad Things Happen to Good People*. New York: Anchor Books, 1981.

Langston, Kelly. *Autism's Hidden Blessings: Discovering God's Promises for Autistic Children & Their Families*. Grand Rapids, MI : Kregel, 2009.

Laugier, Sandra. "The Ethics of Care as a Politics of the Ordinary." *New Literary History* 46, no. 2 (Spring 2015): 217–40.

Lee, Marie Myung-Ok. "Jerry Seinfeld's Not Helping: Celebrity Autism Claims Distract from Reality and Research. Salon, November 10, 2014. https://www.salon.com/2014/11/10/jerry_seinfelds_not_helping_celebrities_with_autism_distract_from_reality_and_research/.

Locke, John. *Essay Concerning Human Understanding*. London: Dent, 1961.

Lord, Catherine, Eva Petkova, Vanessa Hus, Weijin Gan, Feihan Lu, Donna M. Martin, Opal Ousley, Lisa Guy, Raphael Bernier, Jennifer Gerdts, Molly Algermissen, Agnes Whitaker, James S. Sutcliffe, Zachary Warren, Ami Klin, Celine Saulnier, Ellen Hanson, Rachel Hundley, Judith Piggot, Eric Fombonne, Mandy Steiman, Judith Miles, Stephen M. Kanne, Robin P. Goin-Kochel, Sarika U. Peters, Edwin H. Cook, Stephen Guter, Jennifer Tjernagel, Lee Anne Green-Snyder, Somer Bishop, Amy Esler, Katherine Gotham, Rhiannon Luyster, Fiona Miller, Jennifer Olson, Jennifer Richler and Susan Risi. "A Multisite Study of the Clinical Diagnoses of Different Autism Spectrum Disorders." *Archives of General Psychiatry* 69, no. 3 (March 2012): 306–13.

Love, Heather. "Autistic Boy Thrown Out of Public Gardens for His Disability." YouTube, April 5, 2017. https://www.youtube.com/watch?v=Hsria6IFWXM.

Lupkin, Sydney, and Emily Shapiro. "Mom of Girl with Autism Who Was Kicked off Plane Speaks Out." ABC News, May 11, 2015. http://abcnews.go.com/Health/mom-autistic-girl-kicked-off-plane-speaks/story?id=30965376.

Luterman, Sara. "Autistic Advocates Clash with Autism Parents at Government Committee Meeting." *NOS Magazine*, October 27, 2017. http://nosmag.org/parents-and-autistic-adults-clash-at-autism-committee-meeting-iacc-interagency-autism-coordinating-committee/.

Lutz, Amy S. F. "Dear Stranger: Your Son's Autistic, Just Like Mine." Babble, September 13, 2007. https://www.babble.com/toddler/talking-to-parents-of-autistic-children-signs-of-autism-in-toddlers/.

174   *Bibliography*

———. *Each Day I Like It Better: Autism, ECT, and the Treatment of Our Most Impaired Children*. Nashville: Vanderbilt University Press, 2014.

———. "Friends for Hire? For Those with Severe I/DD, Relationships with Direct Care Staff Are Primary." *Psychology Today*, October 14, 2018. https://www.psychologytoday.com/us/blog/inspectrum/201810/friends-hire.

———. "Who Decides Where Autistic Adults Live?" *The Atlantic*, May 26, 2015. https://www.theatlantic.com/health/archive/2015/05/who-decides-where-autistic-adults-live/393455/.

May, Ted, dir. *Elmo's World: Dancing, Music, Books*. 1999; Burbank, CA: Warner Brothers Studio, 2020. DVD.

Mazurek, Micah, Stephen Kanne, and Ericka Wodka. "Physical Aggression in Children and Adolescents with Autism Spectrum Disorders." *Research in Autism Spectrum Disorders* 7, no. 3 (March 2013): 455–65.

McMahon, Jeff. *The Ethics of Killing: Problems at the Margins of Life*. Oxford: Oxford University Press, 2002.

Mead, Kit. "How the Media and Society Objectify Disabled People." *Paginated Thoughts* (blog), September 5, 2016. https://kpagination.wordpress.com/2016/09/05/how-media-and-society-objectify-disabled-people/.

Medina, Kathy. *Finding God in Autism: A 40 Day Devotional for Parents of Autistic Spectrum Children*. Mustang, OK: Tate, 2006.

Meier, Madeline H., Avshalom Caspi, Antony Ambler, HonaLee Harrington, Renate Houts, Richard S. E. Keefe, Kay McDonald, Aimee Ward, Richie Poulton and Terrie E. Moffitt. "Persistent Cannabis Users Show Neuropsychological Decline from Childhood to Midlife." *Proceedings of the National Academy of Sciences* 109, no. 40 (October 2, 2012). http://www.pnas.org/content/109/40/E2657/tab-article-info.

"Minnesota Mom Charged for Treating Son's Pain with Medical Marijuana." CBS News, August 21, 2014. https://www.cbsnews.com/news/minnesota-mom-charged-for-treating-sons-pain-with-medical-marijuana/.

Montaigne, Michel de. "Of Friendship." In *Works of Michel de Montaigne: Comprising His Essays, Journey into Italy, and Letters*. Edited by William Hazlitt, 264–81. Boston: Houghton, Osgood and Company, 1879.

Moore, G. E. *Principia Ethica*. Cambridge: Cambridge University Press, 1903.

National Council on Disability. "NCD Policy Areas," accessed December 2, 2018. https://ncd.gov/.

National Council on Severe Autism. "Frequently Asked Questions," accessed August 29, 2019. https://www.ncsautism.org/faqs.

Nehamas, Alexander. *On Friendship*. New York: Basic Books, 2016.

The New Testament in Modern English. Translated by J. B. Phillips. New York, NY: Macmillan Publishing Co., Inc., 1958.

Nichols, Mike, dir. *Regarding Henry*. 1991; Hollywood, CA: Paramount Pictures.

Padgett, Jason, and Maureen Seaberg. *Struck by Genius: How a Brain Injury Made Me a Mathematical Marvel*. Boston: Houghton Mifflin, 2014.

Patterson, Meagan M., and Rebecca S. Bigler. "Preschool Children's Attention to Environmental Messages about Groups: Social Categorization and the Origins of Intergroup Bias." *Child Development* 77 (2006): 847–60.

Perry, David M. "How 'Inspiration Porn' Reporting Objectifies People with Disabilities." Medium, February 25, 2016. https://medium.com/the-establishment/how-inspiration-porn-reporting-objectifies-people-with-disabilities-db30023e3d2b.

Pinker, Steven. *The Blank Slate: The Modern Denial of Human Nature*. New York: Penguin Books, 2002.

Pyle, Rod. "Probing the Mysterious Perceptual World of Autism." California Institute of Technology, October 22, 2015. http://www.caltech.edu/news/probing-mysterious-perceptual-world-autism-48543.

Querry, K. "Heartwarming Promposal: Cheerleader Asks Boy with Autism to Prom." Oklahoma's News 4. February 23, 2016. http://kfor.com/2016/02/23/heartwarming-promposal-cheerleader-asks-boy-with-autism-to-prom/.

Rahman, Khaleda. "Mother of Autistic Boy Says She Was Humiliated after They Were Kicked Out of Pizza Restaurant Because He Was Being 'Too Loud.'" *Daily Mail*, October 9, 2016. http://www.dailymail.co.uk/news/article-3829500/Mother-autistic-boy-says-kicked-pizza-restaurant.html.

Raine, Adrian. *The Anatomy of Violence: The Biological Roots of Crime*. New York: Pantheon Books, 2013.

Rosa, Shannon Des Roches. "*Rolling Stone*: Your Dehumanization of Autistic People Is the Problem." *Squidalicious* (blog), July 27, 2016. http://www.squidalicious.com/2016/07/rolling-stone-your-dehumanization-of.html.

Ryle, Gilbert. *The Concept of Mind*. Chicago, IL: University of Chicago Press, 2000.

Schofield, Michael. *January First*. New York: Crown, 2012.

Schwarz, Alan. *ADHD Nation: Children, Doctors, Big Pharma, and the Making of an American Epidemic*. New York: Scribner, 2016.

Selman, Robert L. *The Growth of Interpersonal Understanding: Developmental and Clinical Analyses*. New York: Academic Press, 1980.

Singer, Peter. "All Animals Are Equal." In *Animal Rights and Human Obligations*, ed. Tom Regan and Peter Singer. Upper Saddle River, NJ: Prentice-Hall, 1989.

———. *The Expanding Circle: Ethics, Evolution, and Moral Progress*. Princeton, NJ: Princeton University Press, 1981.

Singh, Ilina. "Not Robots: Children's Perspectives on Authenticity, Moral Agency and Stimulant Drug Treatments." *Journal of Medical Ethics* 39,

no. 6 (August 28, 2012).   http://jme.bmj.com/content/early/2012/08/27/
medethics-2011-100224.

Sisti, D. A., A. G. Segal, and E. J. Emanuel. "Improving Long-Term Psychiatric
Care: Bring Back the Asylum." *Journal of the American Medical Association*
313, no. 3 (2015): 243–44.

Solomon, Andrew. "The Autism Rights Movement." *New York*, May 25, 2008.
http://nymag.com/news/features/47225/.

Solotaroff, Paul. "Luke's Best Chance: One Man's Fight for His Autistic Son." *Rolling Stone*, July 27, 2016. https://www.rollingstone.com/
culture/culture-features/lukes-best-chance-one-mans-fight-for-his-
autistic-son-93049/.

Spencer, Liz, and Ray Pahl. *Rethinking Friendship: Hidden Solidarities Today.*
Princeton, NJ: Princeton University Press, 2006.

Stone, Jon, dir. *The Best of Ernie and Bert.* 1998; Los Angeles, CA: Random
House Home Video, 2003. DVD.

Stout, A. "5 Reasons Why Your Child with Autism Needs to Be Out in Public."
The Autism Site, accessed February 10, 2017.   http://blog.theautismsite.
com/seen-in-public/.

Tajfel, Henri. "Experiments in Intergroup Discrimination." *Scientific American* 223, no. 5 (November 1970): 96–103.

Tanakh: The Holy Scriptures. Philadelphia: The Jewish Publication Society, 1988.

Thomson, Donna. "Can Paid Caregivers Also Be Friends?" Dugan Disability
Law, accessed December 18, 2018.

"Toward Autonomy and Self-Determination—World Autism Awareness
Day 2017." UN Web TV, March 31, 2017. http://webtv.un.org/search/
toward-autonomy-and-self-determination-world-autism-awareness-
day-2017/5380816054001.

Tronto, Joan. *Caring Democracy: Markets, Equality, and Justice.* New York:
New York University Press, 2013.

Trousdale, Gary and Kirk Wise, dirs. *Beauty and the Beast.* 1991; Burbank,
CA: Walt Disney Studios, 1994. DVD.

Tsai, Luke Y. "Asperger's Disorder Will Be Back." *Journal of Autism and Developmental Disorders* 43 (2013): 2914–42.

United Nations. "Universal Declaration of Human Rights," 2015, https://
www.un.org/en/udhrbook/pdf/udhr_booklet_en_web.pdf.

US Department of Health and Human Services. *Facing Addiction in America: The Surgeon General's Report on Alcohol, Drugs, and Health.* November 2016. https://www.ncbi.nlm.nih.gov/books/NBK424847/.

Valenti-Hein, Denise, and Linda Schwartz. The Sexual Abuse Interview for Those
with Developmental Disabilities. Santa Barbara, CA: James Stanfield, 1995.

Van Allen, Amanda. "Crying Child with Autism Kicked Out of Restaurant." 69 News, October 12, 2016. http://www.wfmz.com/news/southeastern-pa/crying-child-with-autism-kicked-out-of-restaurant_20161028031651547/133772765.

Vernon, Mark. *The Meaning of Friendship*. Basingstoke: Palgrave Macmillan, 2010.

Volokh, Eugene. "Duty to Rescue/Report Statutes." *The Volokh Conspiracy* (blog), November 3, 2009. http://volokh.com/2009/11/03/duty-to-rescuereport-statutes/.

Waters, Larry J. "Suffering in the Book of Job." In Waters and Zuck, *Why, O God?*, 111–25.

Waters, Larry J., and Roy B. Zuck, eds. *Why, O God? Suffering and Disability in the Bible and Church*. Wheaton, IL: Crossway, 2011.

Wedge, Marilyn. *Suffer the Children: The Case against Labeling and Medicating and an Effective Alternative*. New York: W. W. Norton, 2011.

Wendell, Susan. *The Rejected Body: Feminist Philosophical Reflections on Disability*. New York: Routledge, 1996.

Williams, David. "Undefeated Wrestler Lets Opponent with Down Syndrome Win." CNN, January 28, 2016. http://www.cnn.com/2016/01/28/us/undefeated-wrestler-down-syndrome-irpt/index.html.

Willingham, Emily. "*Rolling Stone* Offers Its Entry Into Parents-First Disability Genre." *Forbes*, July 27, 2016. https://www.forbes.com/sites/emilywillingham/2016/07/27/rolling-stone-offers-entry-into-parents-first-disability-genre/#3d699ec15bdf.

Wilson, Edward O. *The Meaning of Human Existence*. New York: Liveright, 2014.

Wolf, Tom. "Executive Order: 2016-03: Establishing 'Employment First' Policy and Increasing Competitive Integrated Employment for Pennsylvanians with a Disability." March 10, 2016. https://www.governor.pa.gov/newsroom/executive-order-2016-03-establishing-employment-first-policy-increasing-competitive-integrated-employment-pennsylvanians-disability/.

Wyatt, John. "What Is a Person?" *Nucleus*, Spring 2004: 10–15.

Young, Iris Marion. "Asymmetrical Reciprocity: On Moral Respect, Wonder, and Enlarged Thought." *Constellations* 3, no. 3 (1997): 340–63.

Zaslow, Alexandra. "Walmart Employee Gives Shoes off His Feet to Barefoot Homeless Man." *Today*, August 3, 2016. https://www.today.com/money/walmart-employee-gives-shoes-his-feet-barefoot-homeless-man-t101446.

Zimbardo, Philip. *The Lucifer Effect: Understanding How Good People Turn Evil*. New York: Random House, 2007.

Zimbardo, Philip G., and Michael R. Leippe. *The Psychology of Attitude Change and Social Influence*. New York: McGraw-Hill, 1991.